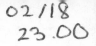

MOTHERS, DAUGHTERS & BODY IMAGE

LEARNING TO LOVE OURSELVES AS WE ARE

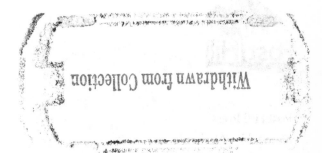

HILLARY L. MCBRIDE

FOREWORD BY DR. RAMANI DURVASULA, PHD

Post Hill
PRESS

A POST HILL PRESS BOOK
ISBN: 978-1-68261-354-2
ISBN (eBook): 978-1-68261-355-9

Mothers, Daughters, and Body Image:
Learning to Love Ourselves as We Are

Cover Image: *En nøgen kvinde sætter sit hår foran et spejl*, by C.W. Eckersberg

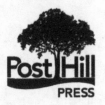

Post Hill Press
New York • Nashville
posthillpress.com

Published in the United States of America

MOMENT ONE

*F*irst moments, the merging of two cells into one, multiplying—two, four, six, eight—rapidly growing and forming the information that will decide my hair, eyes, teeth, hands, my genetic DNA. Everything I needed to become a human and still I am invisible to the naked eye. I am grown from my Mother's own body, my blood from her blood, my heartbeat from her choice; making her belly swell and her hormones go crazy with rage and want for whip-cream filled donuts at 4am.

My body grows and she puts her hand upon her belly to feel a foot kick her side, the jerk of hiccups, the round of my head. She is proud, proud of her body that is a force, source of life to mine.

I grow. Her body tells her it is time; I come into the world with pain and euphoria as she breaks her beautiful body to give me life. She sees me for the first time, what she has made, and it is good. The intricacies of the human body is something staggering—veins, heart, lungs, synapses, toenails, chemicals, eyelashes, all good and beautiful. She holds my body and breathes in.

I grow. From a baby to a toddler, toddler to little girl. I am four and I can run around with my shirt off and feel the fullness of the wind. I can paint my belly and take baths with my friends, slap my butt and laugh. We sleep under stars and run through sprinklers naked and wild. We are silly and think our bodies are strange and wonderful.

I grow and I am six. I am taught what I can and cannot do with my body; can no longer take my shirt off outside on my front porch, no longer run around naked with my friends outside with paint on our bellies because the man across the street stares so my Mother takes me inside and tells me I am now the age where I need to be careful. A feeling comes I never knew before, I learn later the word for it is this—shame. We are at our friend's house and the teenage boy keeps making me sit on his lap; I don't understand it. We are all sitting in a circle, about ten of us, and no one notices. I am confused and try to get away from him, but he holds me there and moves his hands in a way I don't understand. I feel I should obey because he is a strong older boy and I a small girl inherently weaker than he. I get mad that my body is not stronger, that I cannot break free. I feel it is my fault, maybe I should not have worn shorts so my legs were covered. And then there was the church leader, my friend's father, who insisted he put lotion on my legs after our bath. I didn't want him to, but he made me obey, because he was a man, and I, young and born the lesser of the sexes. It is uncomfortable and I thought he must not know what he is doing, a respectable man, let alone a church leader wouldn't do this… but now I am older and know better, yes, he knew. So I am six and I can no longer be free in this body I once ran wild in, but I should cover it because there are predators and I don't tell because I am ashamed, and it was no big deal, no reason to fuss.

I am fourteen. I feel my body changing on me, I notice and others notice and I no longer have the freedom of my youth. Blood comes and I am embarrassed; hiding the grocery store runs, keeping it a secret, seeing my brother laugh when he looks under the sink. It is a wonder of growing to womanhood, but I am starting to hate being a woman. I am ashamed at what my body does, this beautiful thing that I once ran free in is turning on me, making me awkward and uncomfortable because even you are now uncomfortable with that thought. Boy's eyes consume rather than see. I am told this is my fault, I am told God wants me to cover my body, wear longer skirts and shirts up to my collar bone and be sure it isn't tight. But how much skin is okay? Because other girls cover their whole body in black and I heard of the day there were two separate staircases for males and females so that males wouldn't accidentally catch a glimpse of a girl's ankle.

Now that I am fourteen, now that I am changing, is God now ashamed with what he made? The body formed in my mother, so good and beautiful, turned to shame with age and religious threads weaving and constructing my social identity? Oppression for something I cannot control, something completely natural and good. If this body is not holy in and of itself then God should have never made it in the first place. It's the flower hating its vibrant petals, the beautiful tree sprouting from the earth only to grow and be ashamed of its bark.

I am twenty. I have rejected the shy, awkward aspects of womanhood and instead learned to joke about it to cope and be cool. But when night comes, I am often afraid to walk down the street alone. Every walk I take is accompanied with fear, because I see the eyes consume. I hear the threats and am followed. I have friends who are victims. Every girl I know has been afraid, every one of them. From taking a simple walk to rape and a child coming from it. One hid in the laundry basket when she was 9. One silently prayed every night from 13 to 16 that her father would be too drunk to come into her bed. One was at a party with her friend, he wanted something, she didn't, so he trapped her in the restroom. One hid from her brother, another from her grandfather, another from her coworker. Some say it is the woman's fault—the shirt was too low, breasts too big, how can a man resist? But here's a staggering idea: maybe the victim isn't at fault. If in looking at the beautiful woman's body you cannot appreciate her beauty but must strip and consume then it is true our culture has poisoned your mind—consume, take, be the animal, take, take, take.

Shame. Did my mother think that when she held me close to her chest at my birth? Was she ashamed? The beautiful form becomes forbidden and lusted at a certain age, all held together by a story of a serpent and a woman. Though some claim the curse is broken, some still believe it—the body is shamed, curse ever present.

I am thirty. I made two girls within my own body, felt the rush of bringing them into the world, and when I saw their bodies, I saw a miracle. Their skin and eye lashes perfect. Tiny lips, tiny fingernails, eyes embodying innocence and awe. They grow and run around my house naked and scream wildly without self-awareness or social concern. I teach them about our culture and what is and isn't acceptable. But what I will not teach them is shame of their body. It was beautiful from moment one, and that will not change—not with age, not with anything. One daughter looks at her body in the mirror, we talk about the organs and skin, how her body will change. She is beautiful on every count. I remember when I was six, and I know I have to warn her. Not shame her, but tell her how some people were not taught to love, but take for themselves and she must be brave and aware. It pains me as I tell her, her innocent mind not know why one person would hurt another in such a way. "Do not be afraid," I tell her. "But this is our culture, so be smart and be aware my brave girl." Shame teaches us, but I will not teach my daughters in this way. I will empower them to be proud of their bodies, respectful of their bodies, in awe of how miraculous it is and what it is capable of.

I will tell my daughter that to be a woman is not to be lesser, not object, not the bed in the red light district, nor the "bitch" in the hotel. She is not the body to exploit or product to consume.

"She" is not shame.

"She" is beautiful woman with beautiful body, capable of cosmic realities. Holding someone close, experiencing love, making love, creating life, accepting another human life as her own, feeling pain, joy, giving strength, healing with a kiss, wholeness with a touch; giving physical and mental nourishment with her own body.

"She" is grounded enough to follow, still capable to lead from a child to a nation. The woman's body is made in the image of Love, from Love herself, Life herself, so she herself is of God.

For my Grandmother, for my Mother, for my daughters, my friends, and as a reminder to myself: be proud, beautiful woman, your body is intrinsically good, perfectly good.

Perfect from moment one.

Lisa Gungor
gungormusic.com

TABLE OF CONTENTS

Contents

FOREWORD

"**D**oes this make me look fat?"

A reflexive mantra issued by most women, while contorting in front of a mirror.

Most of us are guilty of it, uttering it in front of friends, sisters, retail clerks. A sisterhood of co-conspirators—all of them assuaging us, feeling the same way.

And those of us who are mothers know we have said this in front of our daughters, grimacing once we catch ourselves. A daughter watching in rapt attention as Mommy dresses for work, a night out, or even pulling on her grocery store sweats.

And as with everything else we say and do, they absorb it, and it subtly crafts their developing selves.

Upward of 90 percent of American women are dissatisfied with their bodies. That's a statistic that implies basically every woman in America experiences some level of body dissatisfaction. Where does it come from? All of us are sociologically plugged in enough to know that our perceptions have been altered by the impossible imagery and shaming media. Magazine covers screaming out at us about our abs and our flab, and fetishizing women who gave birth two weeks prior and are back in their "skinny jeans." Seven-year-olds now know how to use photo editing tools to alter their own images—and manipulate themselves into a smaller version of themselves.

But the media is a convenient and perhaps all-too-simple scapegoat. As you are about to discover through the stories of the women you will read, as well as Hillary's story, these narratives go far deeper. They are deeper tales of dissatisfaction, regret, and fear. They are intergenerationally transmitted, like family fairy tales, but these stories also remind us that our narratives are not destiny, that these cycles can be broken. And ultimately they can become tales of empathy, redemption, and love.

I had the pleasure of talking with Hillary about her ideas a few years ago during a chance meeting in Ottawa in a workshop for women in psychology at the Canadian Psychological Association conference. Weight management has been a pivot point in my clinical and research work for years. I have worked with clients who struggle with obesity, disordered eating, and body image distortion. My experience in this space culminated in my first book. But where I learned the most about the importance of narrative on body image was my personal story of weight loss. Much like Hillary, who discovered the nuance of this topic through the brave telling of her own lived experience, it is the miles that we walk ourselves that are often most revelatory. In fact, my legitimacy to my clients did not come from the PhD or the professorship, but rather the fact that I lost 85 pounds and had "before" and "after" pictures to show for it. I personally recognized that health was not just about addressing behaviors and habits but also to look hard at the narratives that shape our health and our habits. This wasn't about protein instead of pastries, or hours in the gym. This was about re-crafting my narrative, and the recognition that health, weight, eating, and body image are an evolving narrative for all women.

Then one day it became *really* personal. When my tween daughter started fretting about body image issues in recent years, my blood chilled. My reflexive defensive maneuver was to blame social media, films, TV, Los Angeles. And then I blamed myself. I sifted through the messages I may have given her. Did she see me vexed over an ill-fitting dress, or ruminating about a slice of cheesecake, or did I let slip a "does this make me look fat?" Because of the nature of my work, I thought I was a relentlessly mindful mother about healthy food, healthy body talk, and regularly taking the time to educate my daughters on how to critically think about the overly sexualized images in the media. Do I turn her into a neo-Luddite and dismiss the phone, the social media, the television? Or do I dig deeper into me, and reach for one of the "ladders" Hillary writes about—to find a new way to have the conversation about body image, a conversation that fits for both my daughters and me? A conversation that takes into account our specific stories, our body shapes, our body types, our lifestyles, our narratives?

We live in the age of "simple solutions"—people want quick fixes and simple palliatives, life advice in 140 characters or less. We want our weight loss advice to be easy and prescriptive—eat this, not that, one-size-fits-all advice. We want to teach girls to be comfortable with their body image, against the backdrop of a photoshopped world, the worship of the ectomorphic, and their mothers' own weight and body fears. But each and every one of us is born into a different family, bringing different stories that shape us (and different body types) and that subsequently shape the worlds of our children.

Rare is the parent who does not want better for her child. Every one of us is aware of the vulnerabilities engendered by our own childhoods, and we vow that we will not repeat those mistakes. We are capable of retelling our stories, but with each generation new vulnerabilities arise, and so too does the aesthetic of a society. Narratives and zeitgeists about body shape and weight may shift with the times. But perhaps our primitive narratives of beauty and being "enough" are ancient stories that lie at the core of these conflicts.

In conducting therapy about weight loss with my clients, if I have learned only one thing, it is that longtime struggles with body image and weight loss are rarely about carbs and runway models. These are complex stories about old hurts, ancient scripts, and sometimes past traumas. Distortions of body image, and dyscontrolled eating, are not simply manifestations of media manipulations or poor willpower, but old narratives that have become so well-worn, they feel like a person's identity. Before my clients know it, the food diaries and exercise goals become conversations about long ago meals at childhood dinner tables, observations of their mothers' regrets, and ultimately letting go of old schemas and personal constructions. Hillary's book highlights the passing down of these old stories, but also how the transformational arc of becoming a parent can force someone to confront these demons in an attempt to avoid passing them down like a dysfunctional familial relic. The next generation can choose to reject these old narratives, and perhaps school their own parents in how to think differently about health and self-value.

We often presume that the body image story is "top-down"—parent teaching child to love her body. But Hillary's book also teaches us that it may be far more reciprocal. Yes, we as parents are the original teachers, and face the responsibilities of teaching our children the fundamentals of healthy nutrition, exercise, and self-care, in addition to the big-ticket psychological scaffolds of attachment, self-regulation, and compassion. But the larger lessons of self-love, authenticity, confidence, and constancy can be quite reciprocal. As our children grow, we are made to face our own fears as parents. The arena in which most of us learn unconditional love happens when we become parents. It may finally be the voices of our children that teach us that we are more than enough, and in turn to accept ourselves and live in a way that models unconditional love—not just for others but also toward ourselves. Our deepest hope must be that this lesson of unconditional love and self-acceptance is paid forward—for our bodies, minds, and lives.

Our narratives are not fixed in stone; they can be re-rendered and revisited. Acceptance is rarely about perfection; it is about compassion. And that may be the most important health message of all.

And perhaps the whole enterprise is better shared in poetry...

I am larger, better than I thought; I did not know I held so much goodness.

All seems beautiful to me. ...
Whoever denies me, it shall not trouble me;
Whoever accepts me, he or she shall be blessed, and shall bless me.

Walt Whitman

Dr. Ramani Durvasula
Los Angeles, CA

ONE

A DAUGHTER'S LETTER

*"... re-examine all you have been told ... and your very flesh shall be
a great poem and have the richest fluency not only in its words but in
the silent lines of its lips and face and between the lashes of your eyes
and in every motion and joint of your body."*

–WALT WHITMAN

I never blamed my mother for my struggle with an eating disorder,
although I had many opportunities. In some ways, that would have
been the easiest thing to do—to put the responsibility for my pain onto
someone else as a way of making sense of it all. In the mother-blaming
world we live in, it may or may not be hard to believe, but people often
encouraged me to blame my mom. This came out in the subtle and not
so subtle ways that people pressed for an answer to questions of "why."
Why was I suffering? It would have been particularly easy when I was the
most ill, or in years of therapy working towards recovery, or even now as
a therapist and researcher trying to make sense of how body image takes
shape in women. There is something human about wanting to make sense
of pain, of the ugly and messy things in life—I think it makes us feel like
we have more control than we do, and if we just knew enough, we could
change it for someone else, for ourselves, for the world. Or, if it's someone

1

else's fault, we are off the hook, and we don't have to examine thoughtfully, painfully, our role in the origin or expression of the suffering.

If I press myself to really think and confess, there were moments when I wanted to, or tried to, blame my mother. But these moments were a long time ago, and didn't usually last for more than a few seconds of frustration, confusion, or desperation, wanting someone else to clean up the mess that it felt like my life had become. I just wanted so badly to feel like how I got there, why I was struggling, was someone else's fault. I didn't believe it was entirely my own, but if not mine, then whose? But the more I thought about it, it didn't make sense to me to put all the responsibility for my pain on her shoulders, when I wouldn't put all the glory for my recovery on her either. Something about that equation didn't make sense. Plus, I couldn't fight the thing that has never felt most true— the thing that has always been most certain for me in my entire life—that my mother loves me more than anything; she wants the best for me, and wants even more for me than she has ever wanted for herself.

When we as therapists and researchers who study body image start to look at understanding young girls' and women's body image problems, it becomes a game of pointing the finger. Surely a struggle which almost every woman experiences must be related to the other experience most women know: having a mother. Finding the space between blaming mothers, and understanding the absolutely sacred and essential role they have in raising their daughters, is like walking a very delicate tightrope suspended between two impossibly tall buildings: balance is everything. Mothers are the most dynamic and influential force on the development of a young woman's journey to being herself. This will ultimately be one of the most defining relationships of her life, and probably her first real encounter with love. And, this sacred relationship will most likely also be her first deep encounter with struggle and pain, as a daughter learns to push against her mother to find out who she is as an individual. The problem is that the story often ends there, when there is really so much more than the pushing away, blaming, and hurt. Mothers have the power to be the most important person in helping their daughters know freedom, voice, depth, beauty, power, and safety.

Most of us have spent our entire lives learning about, then perfecting, the performance of the role of the "good woman." We have learned that as a woman it is best to be quiet, to be sweet, small, and compliant, and to keep working on the "project" of our bodies to make them look more and more desirable. Even though I've made peace with my story, and the road it took to get where I am now, there are still a few things I can't, and refuse, to let go of. As women, rarely do we know what it looks, feels, or sounds like to ourselves as we are. I've worked hard to piece together stories and relationships in my own life that have helped me have something—a vision, a narrative—of what it means to be a woman in this world. I have met several women, and am blessed to have deep friendships with women who love their bodies (and themselves) as they are. They are the proof of victory, the beacon of hope for myself and for other women. But, their experiences aren't the normal experiences for most women. In fact, whenever I talk about "women loving their bodies," most teen and adult women say "that's not possible" or "that's not the whole truth." These responses identify the problem that I can't, and won't, let go of: if as women we don't believe it's possible to love our bodies as they are, how are we going to find the courage to carve that path on our own? How can we work for and build something we don't believe can exist? How can we love ourselves, our bodies, and each other as we are?

"WHAT WENT RIGHT?"

We don't hear very often the stories when it comes to women's relationships to their bodies when things "go right," and what happened along the way that helped these women get there. This is true both in the public (think news, print media, and social media) and in academic and therapeutic settings (in psychology we have had a long history of researching people who have mental illness, not mental health). I have heard countless stories of women, as a therapist, researcher, and friend, who've come back from a vicious battle with body-shame and won. Yet, I started to wonder—what happens when women skip that "I hate my body and want to cut off my thighs" phase, and jump right to the "I don't look like women in magazines and shouldn't, and love myself just as I am" phase? And, what might mothers have to do with all of that?

I can make it sound like I was trying all along to write the book you hold within your hands. The truth is that the research I've done for this book was because I had some questions I wanted to ask, motivated by my own deep fear. I desperately want to understand how to help a daughter love her body, right from the get-go, because I want to have a daughter one day. And, I want to know I did everything I could, in spite of my own wounds, to give her the best shot that I can in this confusing, mysterious, wonderful, and often painful world. I want to do everything I can to protect her, and every other woman, from struggling in the same way I did. So, I set out to find a group of young women who had never had an eating disorder, and really, truly, deep-down loved themselves. I wanted to hear their stories of struggle and strength, and I was deeply curious to learn what their mothers did, and didn't do, so that I could learn from their wisdom. In the process, I was transformed in more ways than I could have imagined. I started talking about what I was finding out in the research to my friends, my clients, other researchers and academics, and women everywhere wanted to talk about it too. And they didn't want just the abbreviated version, they wanted the real stories, the honest words, the hopeful truths. It turns out that as women, there is a lot of us who want to know that there is another way to live besides being constantly bombarded with thoughts about how bad you look, and how ashamed you are of your body. It also turns out that the things I found out from these young women, and their mothers, hadn't been talked about before. The more we talked about it with each other, and shared our insights with other women, we started to believe as women that "another way" was really possible.

But, we can't do it alone—and I don't believe we were ever meant to. In fact, what was so unique about the story of the development of these women's healthy body image was the role that relationship played in it all. That's where the mother part comes in. If mothers really are as influential as we say they are, then they have the potential, through relationship with their daughters, to protect their daughters, to fight for them, to create a new world for them, and give them freedom (not just baggage). The best news of all is that this can happen even when mothers are still struggling in their own journey to love their bodies. That means that no matter where you are right now in your life, in your struggle to fight with or love your body, you can be part of creating change for the women who are coming after you. And, you don't have to stop it there. By being part of a movement to help all women—and your daughter, if you have one—love themselves in their bodies, you'll start to experience this for yourself too. This is for me and most other women who read this the most liberating part of what you're going to be reading: you don't have to be perfect to help change things in your daughter's life, in your community, and in the world. In fact, what the world of young and not-so-young women needs is to see other women who, in spite of being imperfect, are a powerful force to be reckoned with.

In the process of doing all the work of finding these amazing women and hearing their stories, I knew that I was going to look at ways my mother had shaped me. I would have to acknowledge all the ways she had helped me become me. This meant looking past all the stuff I don't like that I "inherited" from her. These were, and still are, my mother's greatest gifts to me: her love, the opportunity to let me think for myself—even when it hurt her—and the tenacious spirit to fight for justice.

No woman is perfect, no mother is perfect. But we each have something very special to offer each other. I hope that in reading this book you will be inspired to notice and share these gifts with your daughter and the other women around you. This is not the kind of "inspired" in the

"I-have-jeans-two-sizes-too-small-in-my-closet" sense of the word, but in its truest form—that you believe that it's possible as girls and women, as daughters and mothers, to love ourselves just as we are.

TWO

THE LADDER OUT: STANDING ON HER SHOULDERS

"I once dreamt I was telling stories and felt someone patting my foot in encouragement. I looked down and saw that I was standing on the shoulders of an older woman who was steadying my ankles and smiling up at me.

I said to her, "no no come stand on my shoulders, For you are old and I am Young."

"No no" she insisted, "this is the way it is supposed to be." I saw that she stood on the shoulders of a woman far older than she, who stood on the shoulders of a woman even older, who stood on the shoulders of a woman in robes, who stood on the shoulders of another soul, who stood on the shoulders..."

–CLARISSA PINKOLA ESTÉS,
Women Who Run With The Wolves

It happened today, again. I have these moments every so often when I realize with simultaneous amusement and terror that I am becoming my mother. I was late for an important meeting, sitting at a standstill in traffic on a busy highway—with apparently nothing to do but become awakened to the subconscious patterns of my family of origin. There is this thing that my mom has always done: in her car she sets the clock 15 minutes ahead to help herself get somewhere on time. The thing that happens when she does this, though, is that she always remembers that the clock is 15 minutes fast, so the trick doesn't work and she gets places at the same time she always would. In my adulthood I've realized my own version of the "car-clock" trick—my watch is usually fast by five minutes. And today as I was sitting in my car, nowhere near the destination I was supposed to be five minutes earlier, I realized I had fallen for the same trick. In no way had setting my watch a few minutes faster gotten me out of the house earlier than I would have normally. I just look at my watch, knowing it is fast, and think, "I've got time."

Gasp. No one was twisting my arm—*it was me who did this*. I've had more experiences with this too—making big batches of soup on Sundays for meals in the coming week, carrying too many bags from the car so I only have to make one trip, assembling the same kind of tomato sandwich in the exact same way that she does when I need a meal in a pinch, and so many more. As it turns out, there is a word for this fear: matrophobia. That is the official word for the dread of becoming one's mother. After laughing with delight at the word itself, I took comfort in knowing that this was something so common there is actually a word for it. It is a normal, if not entirely universal, fear that we will one day become our mothers. We can adore them, appreciate their generosity and unconditional love, and still be struck with terror at realizing that our efforts to push against their annoying idiosyncrasies to be a totally different and unique person were futile, and we are more alike than not.

This is one of the fears I hear from mothers most when they're coming in for therapy. It doesn't usually come out right away, but at some point in the process of doing therapy a woman will want to do some work about how to be different than her mother. Not just her fear of taking on her mother's little mannerisms, but of hurting her children, her daughter, in the way her mother hurt her or let her down.

ALL THE DROPS COUNT

Even though all our stories as women are different, we all have a story of how we became who we are. And whether we like it or not, that story is usually shaped at least in some ways by our mother (whether she was physically or emotionally present, or not). This may feel scary to think about, both as you think about who you are, and who your daughter may become, but I want to remind you that no matter what anyone says, life isn't as deterministic we are often told. What we think and want and do matters: we are not just the sum of the mistakes that our mothers made, or the mistakes we have made up until this moment. Who we are in this moment, and who we are working to become, also counts for something; we and our daughters can be more than our accidents, mess-ups, and fears.

At a certain moment in our lives we get the opportunity to make some choices about what we do with that story of how we became the self we are today. Having a daughter is special, in that you get opportunities every day to make those choices. There are the big moments, like the screaming-at-each-other-fight, where it seems easy to identify that in that moment you can do something different than your mother might have done for you. But we forget that there are also hundreds of little moments that make up our day when we can make small choices to do something differently than how our mothers before us did. Those small moments, like how you respond when your child walks in the door after school, when she asks for a snack, or what you say about something that to you might seem insignificant, but to her might mean the world. When we add up all those millions of small moments, they amount to so much more. Think of these moments like making very small but regular deposits into a savings account—you likely won't notice that a few dollars have been put away, but pretty soon it's added up to something much bigger.

I usually see this going one of two ways: staying stuck, or something I'll call "choosing the ladder." When we are stuck, as individuals or as parents, we recreate the patterns we experienced with our mother internally, and in our relationships with others, especially our daughters. This often happens when a mom is afraid to examine these patterns, or unaware that they exist, and so unknowingly relives them, not ever knowing or working towards another way of being. Most of us fall into this category, even though we may desperately want more for ourselves and for daughters than anyone will ever know. And, this isn't because we are bad, or weak, or unlovable; but sometimes looking backwards, then moving forwards, is a demanding, difficult, and terrifying thing to do.

The other option, "choosing the ladder," is what we saw in the mothers and daughters in this study. The ladder these mothers chose, or what we called it in the study "standing on my shoulders," was our way of saying that the mother could identify and name the negative cycles she had with her own mother, and took deliberate steps to do things differently in her own life, and for her daughter. This didn't mean she was perfect, or did it flawlessly every time, but she wasn't pretending those patterns weren't there, and was passionate about protecting her daughter from her own struggles. In doing so, she offered her daughter a ladder out of her own struggles as woman, into a bigger, brighter, freer world. Although they never expected this, the mothers in the study were transformed in the process of helping to transform their girls. They felt there was meaning in their efforts, and that it was healing for them in their own story to know they broke a cycle that could have gone on indefinitely.

What was really special about these moms was that they didn't just try and protect their daughters from the painful "mother-daughter" relationship wounds, but also from their own individual struggles: like anxiety, depression, or shame. These mothers were able to look at their lives with honesty and courage, and name the things that they had struggled with most. Then they worked hard, in small and big ways, to try to create the opposite experience for their daughters. For example, one of the mothers, Sheree (who you'll meet in a later chapter), has struggled a lot with anxiety. It had shown up in her life in a variety of ways, some more subtle, others more overwhelming and disabling. She actually carried a lot of shame about her struggles at first. But, instead of hiding her struggles, or ignoring that anxiety existed in life, she decided she wanted to talk openly with her daughter about anxiety in general, and reminded all of her kids it was ok to share their feelings with her. Sheree wanted her daughter to know that if she was anxious, she could tell her mother about it, and that she wouldn't be alone.

ANNE'S STORY

This is where I want to introduce some of the women we studied, Kelsey and her mother, Anne, to explain more about how all of the things I'm talking about look in real life. My hope with this is that the ideas I'm talking about will start to come to life, and feel more within your reach. I hope you learn from these women, in ways that I did. And, that you're surprised by how much more you have to offer the world, your daughter, than you originally thought.

Meet Anne. Anne is the middle-aged mother of three who is tall and has a strong voice and deep laugh. I met Anne because her daughter Kelsey was participating in the study—I knew Kelsey loved her body and all other parts of herself (that was assessed quantitatively and qualitatively for inclusion in this specific study). I wanted to know how Anne helped Kelsey love her body, and what she did and didn't do to help Kelsey grow up to be strong, confident, and beautiful—all at the same time. When Anne speaks about her experience of growing up, the story is one of insecurity, pain, and silence. She talked about being insecure because she was taller than other kids her age, and noticing early on that she was different from them because of her height. In our interview, she called her younger self "an ugly duckling," which was a name she was called as a kid. In spite of this, she describes experiencing some of her own physical and mental strength early on through playing sports. Playing on many sports teams as a child helped her feel strong and healthy, and being on a team gave her the chance to feel like she belonged. Although playing sports was helpful, it wasn't enough to help her overcome her insecurity in her appearance—an insecurity that runs from early in her childhood into how she still sees herself now. Although the things that made her insecure as a kid are now gone, age and menopause have come with new challenges that make her feel at odds with her body. She says she's put on more weight, and that her body isn't "cooperating the way it used to."

Although we were just meeting for the first time when I interviewed her, Anne was quite free with how she spoke about herself; she was really honest with how things were in the past and how they are now. Despite the struggles she's having with her appearance now, she says she wants to work on how she feels about herself, about her body. She says about herself-image, "I think it could improve, I think that I need to work a little harder on accepting myself where I am right now, instead of going 'ugh' when I look at myself in the mirror." When listening to Anne speak, this was my first moment of hope about what I can bring to the world, and a future daughter: Her daughter Kelsey was thriving, and confident in herself, which had happened even though Anne still considered her journey of self-acceptance to be a work in progress. What she did do was offer her daughters a ladder: she was aware of how dissatisfied she was with her own body, and wanted to instill in her three daughters that they were beautiful—something she never heard from her own mom. I was so struck by Anne's self-awareness and self-compassion: she realized that she didn't love her body as much as she could, and she realized that was something she wanted to work on. But, she didn't beat herself up about the things she didn't do perfectly. She had a comfortable way of saying that she was working towards loving herself more. Her relationship with her body reminds me of how so many people I know describe their relationships with their partners: they are able to describe that they love the other person in their imperfections, and want to keep working on building the closeness and affection in their relationship, but they also realize it takes time. This all makes me think about what would happen if I was able to love myself, my body, the parts and the whole, in the way that I love other people? What if as women we could dedicate ourselves to practice kindness and care towards ourselves in the way that we are often so good at being kind and caring to those around us?

Anne's desire to give her daughters a "ladder" showed up in many dimensions of their relationships, not just in what she told them about their appearances. She was courageous to believe in, and then act on, the desire to be a better mother to her daughters than her mother was to her. In order to better understand what that meant, I asked her to describe what her relationship with her mom was like growing up. She was quiet for a long time and then said, "With my mother, it was not a close relationship at all. My mom had a very difficult life. ... My mom consequently was very silent and withdrawn. She was just trying to cope, and so we never talked about feelings or thoughts or anything like that. She was kind to me, but it was never more than that.." Listening to Anne's story reveals how what we say is often just as important as what we don't say. We can communicate literally about bodies and say things to other people like "women's bodies are so attractive when they are thin or young," or we can communicate about women's bodies by what we don't say. The silence on certain issues, especially if they are intentionally avoided or dismissed, can communicate to others "this isn't important" or "we don't talk about sex or bodies in our family." Anne says that her mom never spoke to her about bodies, sexuality, or beauty, but instead was focused more on doing tasks, and keeping the house running. Unlike Anne's mom, who was emotionally absent but kind, Anne's dad was abusive towards her in several ways. Anne never told her mother about the abuse. When I asked her about this now, she said that she thinks she was trying to protect her mom from hurting more in her life. When she was saying this, she paused, took a breath and said in a very matter of fact way, "I think deep down I knew that my mom would not do what I [needed] her to, and I think I was trying to protect myself from being totally crushed by that."

13

She found out when she was older that her intuition during those difficult years was right: when she told her mom about it years later she found out that her mother knew all along but never did anything. She courageously confronted her mother about this, and said that her mother "had no good reason" for not sticking up for Anne. When I asked her how this shaped her, she said that all of what she has been through, both the abuse from her dad and knowing that her mother couldn't defend her, made it very hard for her to love and accept herself. That because of this, from early on she worked so hard to try to be as perfect as she could be, thinking that if she was perfect that she might be more loved and accepted. Anne thinks that all of this has been what made it, and still makes it, hard to really accept how she looks—even today.

When she described this difficult confrontation with her mother, I could only imagine the amount of tension they each must have felt. And, through how she described it, I got a profound glimpse into how alone in her life she must have felt for so long. Her mother was there, but not there. Her mother loved her, but never protected or defended her.

As we kept talking, Anne remembered the few things her mother ever said about her own body, and that she wasn't totally silent. Her mom would say things like, "I wish I could get rid of this stomach." What sticks out to me about Anne's story is that in spite of her mother's silence about the abuse, her mother was still able to be vocal about her own body shame. Their relationship, like so many mother-daughter relationships, is one of contradictions and complex ironies. And I believe that these contradictions are related, and tell a story about what it is like to be us on the inside. Some things are too terrifying to name, but other things, often our displeasure with ourselves and our bodies as women, flow freely from our lips.

But, Anne made a choice. She chose to be fierce and to do her best to change the way she lived out the mother-daughter relationship so that she didn't hurt her daughters in the ways her mother hurt her. She worked hard to be more emotionally present, vocal, and active in Kelsey's life. She spoke a lot with me about being intentional about helping Kelsey feel loved, secure, and protected, in ways that her own mother was never able to. When I asked her about the messages she might have communicated to Kelsey about bodies, beauty, and womanhood, she acknowledges that she was probably critical of herself in front of Kelsey. Although she struggled to remember, there were times when she remembers saying things like, "I have nothing nice to wear, this [outfit] doesn't look good," or her recent frustration to find clothes that fit her well so that she likes her body as it is changing through menopause. When I asked Anne about what she might have communicated to her kids without trying, she became quite tentative and said that she always took pride in her appearance and might have communicated to Kelsey that "women should look a certain way," and that it was not good to be seen out in sweatpants, that as a woman "you can't let yourself go…."

Remember what I was saying earlier about not having to do it all perfectly, but about being good enough? The way Anne parented Kelsey is a lot like that. She isn't a fitness guru, she made some "mistakes" too with what she said, and did, that sent Kelsey contradictory messages about bodies and being a woman in this world. And Kelsey still grew up to love herself just as she is. Anne did, however, work hard to be different than her own mother, in how she parented. She said, "Because I always felt like such an ugly duckling when I was young, I always tried to let my kids know that I thought they were beautiful, and they are…."

Towards the end of the interview, I asked Anne what it was like telling me about her story growing up, and how life is now with Kelsey. She said she felt sad "a little bit with [talking about] my mom. It's just that, it's sad for me. … I feel sorry for her, her upbringing, her marriage, and really sad that she didn't have the inner strength to change." This didn't strike me as a pity kind of sadness, but as a kind of empathy for her mother in which she saw and felt her mother's pain as a woman. What she said was quite profound: she wasn't sad for herself anymore, but was sad that her mom would never know the strength she knew. I wasn't quite sure if it was my place to comment on her sadness, but I felt like I couldn't just sit there and not point out the obvious. I saw a woman who had worked hard for a very long time to rewrite the narrative of what it means to be a woman in her family, and in this world. I couldn't help but blurt it out: "You have changed. You've changed, which is powerful. She didn't have the strength to, you did, and you are rewriting the legacy." She seemed hesitant, but relieved to take this in. And we sat in silence for a moment together, just thinking about that. Then she jumped in—"The part that felt cool about [this interview] was remembering that I did try and let my kids know that I thought they were wonderful. ... I do think maybe I could have done more ... but I tried to say that ... it was my goal to communicate that 'you're beautiful no matter what,' so I'm hoping that part of it is that she felt that she was loved for who she was, not for what she looked like." We smiled at each other, and it seemed to me like a moment of victory that this woman who had come from a childhood of abuse and aloneness is recognizing that even in her imperfection, she has fought hard for her children, and done the best that she can.

KELSEY'S STORY

Listening to Anne speak about her story lit curiosity in me to hear Kelsey's version—I wondered how they each saw each other, and if their perceptions of themselves and the other were overlapping or completely different. The complexity of our relationships to other people ensure that we can both be involved in an interaction, and walk about with different interpretations and explanations of what happened. But with Kelsey and Anne, we knew the punch line—Kelsey is a thriving young woman who loves the space she takes up, and has a healthy relationship with her body. But I wanted to know what happened along the way, and how she felt her mother played a role in her own experience of embodiment. If you were sitting across from Kelsey, you would probably feel very safe and warm all over: she has the kindest, sparkling blue eyes, full of wonder, delight, and a pinch of mischief. When you're with her, she makes it seems like it's finally ok to be yourself, and that being you might really actually be better than being who someone else wants you to be. I think it's because she knows that about herself, and somehow that knowing, and permission for freedom, oozes out of all of her. She is tall like her mom, and is her mother's daughter in many ways—yet also completely her own person. When I asked her to finish the sentence "my body is ..." she said without taking a second to think about it "my body is sacred."

But Kelsey is also honest as she describes that getting to the belief that her body—herself—is sacred was a process. In our interview, she spoke about being aware from a very early age that her tallness might not be considered attractive to boys, and to her that was scary. She told me about being six, and sitting next to her mom in their van, and saying to her mom, "Do you think boys will like me because I'm tall? ... But I'm blonde so maybe they will still like me." In telling me this memory, I could see that at six years old she was already aware of what it meant to be attractive, and how central attractiveness is to so many women She told me another memory about being in kindergarten and at the pool with friends—sucking in her stomach so she would look thinner like another girl who was there. Already in kindergarten she was aware that in our culture being thin is better than being "you" if the "you" is perceived in any way as being "not thin." She had at six been sensitive to the sociocultural messages which inundate our dialogues about what it means to be a girl or woman, and that as women we must be certain things to be desired by men, and being desired by men—as the messaging goes—is the most important thing we can achieve as girls and women. We learn at such early ages now how to compare ourselves to the measuring stick of the images we see in magazines, on runways, and in movies. When we don't "measure up," we are often riddled with shame, and fear. And sometimes burn with determination to move far away from shame, and closer inch by inch, or pound by pound, or meal by meal, towards the measuring stick which tells us we are finally desired, and lovable. Unlike for so many of us, those stories were the exception for Kelsey in a childhood where she was able to play and enjoy the freedom of being a kid. She played sports, and remembers feeling strong in her body, aware of her power and the life within her. For the most part, she had an unassuming relationship with her body which was more about healthy function and play—it was about what her body could do, and not as much that she was her body, and that that was beautiful.

Still, there was more to the story, and as she declared initially, when she spoke about her journey to where she is now, she identified a journey that was not smooth—there were many shifts that occurred within her relationship to her body. The first major shift came after she went through puberty in high school and she started to develop physically. She remembers that she was seen as attractive and that getting attention because of her body felt good. When describing this time of her life she says, "I think I sexualized my body. It garnered me the attention that I felt I needed to gain approval. … I remember wanting my body to be seen as sexy, so that I felt like I was ok." I was so impressed, and still am, by Kelsey's awareness of how she used her body to feel ok about who she was as a person, to feel more valuable. So many of us do this, often without even knowing, or without being critical of it. We treat our bodies like objects, and put them on display, like items strategically presented in a storefront window to draw customers in.

As good as this felt for a time, she seemed to be also aware that it was a feeling that was also hollow. This is the most striking thing about Kelsey's story—that even though she was "using her body" to make herself feel better, and got caught up in objectifying herself for a time, she always has a sense that this was a dead end. That this, chasing the attention men gave her for her body, was never something that would fill her up and make her "whole"– that wholeness and worth needed to come from something other than attention to her appearance. She speaks to this tension when she says, "I liked the attention I received from men, even though I hated it at the same time, so I became very aware of it." I wish Kelsey never felt insecure enough to objectify herself for the emotional reward of attention and affection, but I wish for all of us that we could realize that emptiness of participating in our own objectification to try to ensure our worth. As Kelsey learned, the hollowness of using our bodies in this way continues to trap us, leaving us feeling like we must relentlessly pursue appearance and bodily perfection if we want to keep our "enoughness." It keeps us from seeing that we have so much more to experience in life and offer each other than ceaselessly chasing a carrot, strung by a society that is scared of our greatness as women and will never satisfy us if ever caught.

"I AM ENOUGH."

Things weren't perfect for Kelsey, and the next shift in her journey came when she developed a hormonal imbalance that made her gain weight and get severe acne. It seemed painfully ironic that someone who was getting so much attention for being beautiful all of a sudden had to grapple with the changes happening within her that made her feel so not-beautiful. Her challenges with her new appearance seemed to expose her insecurity underneath—the insecurity that all of her attractiveness in the eyes of others had previously covered up. And because of her forced encounter with her deep insecurity, the struggle with acne and weight gain ultimately led her to experience healing on the deepest level possible. She learned to find her beauty, and value, even when she didn't look the way she believed, and others believed, that she was "supposed to." She describes being in her house, and having a profound spiritual encounter with God which allowed her to realize that her value and worth come from more than how she looks. I still need to pause to take that in. When she told me this story, and even as I write it, it hits me so deeply, and captures something I wish for every woman to experience in her own way. She describes praying in her room one day, her face covered with cystic acne, and says, "I was naked, I had no makeup on, and I looked in the mirror and wrote all over the mirror in marker 'I AM ENOUGH.' " In that moment of rawness and vulnerability, her story shifted again, and she describes finally knowing that her value and sense of self is about more than how she looks. Her body is an important part of who she is, but her appearance doesn't define her worthiness for love and belonging, and she is no less valuable, lovable, or beautiful if she weighs more than our culture tells her she is supposed to. As with her mother's story this story sounds like triumph and bravery over the painful prison of believing we are only choosable if we look a certain way.

I asked her about how the shift that happened in that moment shows up in her life today, and she reflected on taking less time to get ready for the day than she used to, and that she has made the choice to put more energy into the things that she values most, that her appearance isn't the most important thing about her anymore. It was particularly meaningful to me that she hasn't hidden her beauty, but believes that beauty can draw people closer to spirituality, to God, to each other. She doesn't hide that she is striking to look at. She says, "I can still be beautiful, but not let that be my identity, do you know what I mean?" I did, and have so felt that struggle in myself. How can we learn to appreciate and feel our beauty, and the beauty in others, without it defining us? How can we as women learn to appreciate and feel beauty, within others and ourselves, without letting it take away from the other equally important parts of our self?

ANNE'S LADDER TO KELSEY

Remember Anne's story of hurt, her mother's silence, and her desire to do things differently than her mother did? Anne was determined to be more vocal with her daughters. And although it appears she was mostly successful at this, Kelsey still remembers her mother not saying too much about bodies, beauty, weight, and womanhood. Yet, Kelsey always knew her mother believed she was beautiful. Anne wasn't perfect at this, but both Kelsey and Anne believe she was "good enough" at it. Kelsey also knew how strong and courageous her mother was, and how far she had come as a woman in her own struggle. In age-appropriate ways, Anne had told Kelsey about her painful story of growing up, with a courageous honesty that might explain some of Kelsey's freedom to be herself and connect freely with others. Not only had Anne given Kelsey a ladder, but Anne had started to climb it herself. Kelsey talked about wanting to protect her mother; when she had learned to love herself, she wanted the other women in her life to love themselves too. Kelsey encouraged her mother, and reminded her mother of all of the things she had learned in her own journey: she is enough, she is beautiful just as she is, and it is an empty yet tempting path to think we can earn our worth as women through our appearance. When I think about these two women, I think of Anne having given Kelsey a ladder—offering her the opportunity to have a life full of more love, safety, and openness than she had. Then, as Kelsey climbed this ladder, and out of love for her mother, Kelsey reached a hand down to Anne and invited her to climb up as well.

If we look at three generations of women in this family, there is a pattern here between Kelsey and her mother as well: both women worked hard to pull their mothers up their own ladder of growth. The biggest difference between Kelsey and her mother was that Kelsey could acknowledge that she had worth, and that the cultural messages around her (what she saw in magazines and TV) which were describing a life only pursuing attractiveness were hollow and would never fulfill her, or accurately reflect her sacredness. Kelsey can articulate that the sense of emotional safety her mother gave her was an important part of this process—she always felt loved, and accepted by her mom. This safety was something Anne was never able to feel with her own mother, and her mother quite literally did not keep her safe from the abuse. Because she felt so loved and accepted by her mother, just as she was, Kelsey identifies that that helped her love and accept herself. It was as if she had internalized her mother's love.

Anne gave so much to Kelsey—she gave her best. Although it was not perfect, between this mother and daughter there is so much more openness and dialogue than Anne ever had with her mother. Not surprisingly, just like her mother, Kelsey hopes to have a daughter one day who she can give more to than she ever received. She loves her mother, and still acknowledges that there are a few things she was missing. If she were to ever have a daughter, she would want to also give her daughter a ladder of her own. She says, "I'd want to speak so many truths over my daughter's life about her body, and what's expected by society—where her identity and her value lies in, and help her see these things and begin to question them for herself. I think being critical of these messages we're told helps us build resilience."

What I hope for Anne, and every mother, is that she's able to get to where her daughter is one day—to see her own worth, and accept herself as she is. And, I hope this for you too. I wonder what you thought about, and were reminded of, when you read this; if you saw yourself in Kelsey, in Anne, or even in Anne's mother. And I wonder what that inspires you to do.

THE INVITATION TO THE TREE

Imagine that you're in the park in the middle of a city, on a beautiful sunny summer day. And, as beautiful as it is, you can only see so much because all around the park are buildings that shut you off from the horizon. You're standing next to a tree that reaches way up into the sky, and you imagine you could see the wide-open sky much better if you were up in the branches of the tree. But, you're too scared to climb it. You're afraid of heights. Plus, you were told by your mother that "good women don't climb trees." Your daughter is with you in the park, dancing circles around you and doing cartwheels in the grass and daisies. It would be so easy to keep things the way they are, but you remember that your mother was scared of letting you go to the park at all, and yet she gave you the opportunity to do something she was never able to do. Your life was better for it—you saw more of the world, and got to play in a way that your mother was never able to. And, you want your daughter to live in the world in ways that are freer than you were able to, instead of getting stuck carrying your baggage. So you go find a ladder. And maybe it takes a little while, but you bring it back to the park and summon all the courage you can. You steady the ladder, and as you call your daughter over and invite her to climb the tree, you see the sparkle of delight and mischief in her eye. She starts to climb, and you're scared and excited all at the same time. She climbs higher and higher, and squeals with delight, "I can see so much from up here, Mom, it's so beautiful," and then she looks down at you and says, "Will you come up and join me?"

Maybe you are not a mother yet, maybe you have sons, or maybe you're beginning your journey of healing your relationship with your body. You can make many choices in your life about what to do with where you've come from. I dare you to hope and borrow courage from the stories of Kelsey and Anne that you can bring into the world, for those you love most, including yourself, all of the things you deeply needed when you were growing up but never had. I hope you can love yourself and the others in a way that you deserve to feel, because your daughter, the women around you, the world, deserve that too. My hope is in extending this gift of freedom, insight, love, and security that you never had, that you realize that you can have, and deserve, those things too.

REFLECTION QUESTIONS

- What have you struggled with in your life?
- What did you need growing up that you never had?
- If you could give your (current or future) daughter freedom from something that has weighed you down in your life, what would it be?
- What could you do to get out from under that weight?
- What's getting in the way of you being able to help your daughter in the same way?
- What are the hard but important conversations you need to have with your daughter? What about the other women in your life? How might you prepare these conversations so they are honest, yet gentle, and appropriate for the audience with which you desire to share?

- When have you tried, or wanted to, but it hasn't gone well?
- What are some small, daily, ways that you could give her what you never had?

THREE

HONESTY: TELLING THE TRUTH ABOUT WHO WE ARE

"Tear off the mask. Your face is glorious."

–RUMI

One of the great things about being a therapist is hearing how women of all ages and backgrounds speak when they're just being themselves and not worrying about what other people (in this case, me) will think of them. They come into my office, and sometimes right away, other times over many weeks and months, they trust me. And when they trust me, the masks come off. I'm privileged because I get to see women in their most raw and vulnerable forms, without all of the masks we have learned to wear as women. Sometimes these masks look like "perfectionism" and hide that feeling of "if-maybe-I-can-do-this-perfectly-I-won't-feel-like-such-a-failure" underneath. Another mask is the one of kindness to conceal the "I-can't-believe-she-let-her-kid-do-that" thoughts underneath. And the one I see the most: the mask of confidence to cover up the "I-have-no-idea-what-I'm-doing" feeling. We wear masks so much in general that therapy is extra special when it's a mom I'm working with, because the pressure on moms to "appear like they have it all together" is even greater than for anyone else. A mom gets to come into my office and be exactly who she is, in order to explore where she's come from and where she's going.

What usually happens is that we start to explore who she is underneath all of the facades, and she gets really scared. She is afraid that she'll show me her authentic self and I'll judge or reject her. She gets scared that she'll find something she doesn't want to see. Or we discover that she is fundamentally terrified that she'll realize she doesn't actually really like what's underneath the masks after all. But, and this is my favorite part, in the process of therapy she starts to find out that all of that stuff underneath the covering-up is stuff that makes her uniquely her. And, although she was covering it up, it was there all along and she knew that, whether she was acknowledging that to herself or not.

We all wear masks at different times in our lives. Whether we want to admit it or not, they're there. I don't think this is always a bad thing—sometimes wearing a mask is the protection we need. This makes me think about times I've gotten bad news about something, and had to go immediately into an important meeting. In order to be present, to be engaged, and not let all of my feelings about the bad news be written all over my face, I gave myself the best pep talk I could in a bathroom mirror and put on the "I-got-this" mask. I've also worn masks for several years at a time that said "everything's fine," when deep down I was hurting, afraid, and alone.

The problems with these cover-ups start to show up when we don't know when to take them off, or don't know how to take them off. When this happens, we risk living a life that appears one way on the outside, but is totally different on the inside. Or maybe even worse, we risk not ever really learning who we are. We are in danger of holding in all our hurt, or joy, and feeling ultimately alone, isolated, and unsure if we are good enough just as we are. Letting ourselves be seen without covering up by the right people, at the right time, can be one of the most healing things that we do—both for the people who get to see the real us, and for ourselves. When we let ourselves be seen authentically, "warts and all," as the expression goes, not only can we begin to experience acceptance, but we also give other people permission to take off their own masks. When we practice this kind of authenticity in life, we can begin to change the entire meaning of what it means to be a woman. Can you imagine if this were the case? That instead of trying to be a certain kind of version of yourself, you could just be you? Wouldn't it be amazing if "just being you" was something that wasn't only accepted, but was celebrated? And, think about how less alone we would feel as women if instead of competing for some impossible unattainable form of perfection, we shared our struggles—and in doing so could rely on the support of other women who've gone before us, and walked through struggles and came through the other side? And, what if from the very beginning you helped your daughter discover who she is, and love it, so she could cover things up if she needed, but she was fundamentally aware of, and ok with, who she is?

Here's how this all ties into being a mom, and helping your daughter— giving her a ladder, as I described it before. We all think that the masks we put up are convincing, but chances are we're only fooling ourselves. Daughters are wired to be supernaturally perceptive about what their mothers are feeling, doing, and thinking. And in particular, they're highly aware if those messages (what you say, and what you do) match up and are consistent or not. In fact, chances are that she's probably more aware of some of your baggage than you are. So, if we think about the idea of wearing masks in life, and hiding who we really are underneath some kind of cover-up—the reality is that you're probably not hiding it as well as you thought, plus you're also giving your daughter a crash course in learning to be someone she's not. Think about this from your experience as a daughter—you probably remember when your mom was very much "not fine," but when you asked her what was wrong she said, "Nothing, I'm fine."

There is some scary research out there, just in case you think you're fooling anyone. Some researchers have been able to identify that what daughters think (notice and perceive) about what their mothers do to diet, or manage their weight, is important in determining the daughter's own dieting and weight loss attitudes and behaviors.[1] Try reading that again. Try thinking about what you learned from the women around you growing up. This flies in the face of the old expression, do as I say, not as I do. It's more complicated than that. What we believe the other person (in this case, the mother) thinks about bodies and weight is actually incredibly influential. You may not even consciously be aware of what you're actively thinking or feeling about weight loss, but if your daughter thinks that you think that losing weight will make you more beautiful—doesn't matter how she got there—then the chances are that she's going to think that. The evidence that I have seen says that what we think the other people close to us think matters too, but moms are really important.

What's even scarier is that the comments we just let slip out of our mouths without really even thinking that anyone is listening also negatively affect a daughter's dissatisfaction with her own body. For example, you might really want your daughter to believe that she is pretty just as she is, and if you were asked to sit her down and give her a serious talk about body image, that's probably what you'd want to say. And, we think that it's those times when we're trying to be really intentional about communicating something that defines what we're actually communicating. But all those little comments, sighs, and grumblings that we make about our own bodies, those matter too. The things you say matter, even when you're frustrated that your jeans that fit you last year don't fit anymore. When she hears you talk about those things, even when you don't know she hears you, those comments have been shown to actually make her be more likely to dislike her body and try weight loss techniques, even in girls as early as grades 4 to 6.[2] In another study, when mothers made comments, whether on purpose or not, about their own weight and weight loss, this was related to a decrease in her daughter's value of her own body.[3] Imagine you're driving in the car with your daughter, and you say out loud—mostly to yourself—"Oh, I shouldn't have eaten that muffin, now I'm going to feel fat all day." In the study I mentioned above, that comment would actually be felt by your daughter as a direct hit to her ability to appreciate and love her body. This is scary information to realize. If what we do affects other people, shaping who they feel they are and what is valuable about them, then for all of us as women, especially for the developing minds we are nurturing, we need to be careful about what we say about our bodies and each other's bodies. We are relational beings, who grow and develop our identity in relationship to people around us. This ties into Brené Brown's work about shame, and how this deep pain of feeling not good enough can be contagious to those around us. When the people around us carry shame, it can influence the ways we see ourselves. And sadly, when we feel shame, even without knowing it, our shame could bleed into the identities and feelings of others.

Aside from the feeling and experience of shame, some of this also has to do with perception. Perception is complex, and no less complex when it relates to the multilayered relationship between every mother and daughter. I'm sure there are many different things that affect how your daughter interprets what you say about her, and what you say about yourself—like if she believes you, and feels safe with you or not. Think about your own story of growing up and interpreting with your young mind what your mother did and said. You might even have the pleasure and confusion of having grown up with a sibling who heard and saw the same things, but felt differently about them. What is meant to be communicated, and how it is perceived, can often be very different. The scary part about all this research is that even the things moms don't mean for their daughters to hear, or don't mean for their daughters to take as seriously about herself, do in fact affect her. Knowing this demands hope. Fortunately, hope is obvious in the stories of the women who were interviewed.

What showed up when we interviewed the young women and their moms is that most of the moms weren't totally thrilled about how they looked and tried to hide it from their daughters. Mothers are always surprised by this one, but the daughters in us never are: even what the moms thought they hid, the daughters knew anyway. Seeing this in their moms hurt the daughters. It made them feel sad for themselves, and start to doubt themselves, and mistrust their mothers for not telling them the truth. It also made them feel sad for their mothers, and want to protect and take care of their mothers. The difficult balance here, another tightrope to walk, is how to find the space of honesty without hiding who you are and what's going on and showing her so much of your story that she feels it is her job to take care of you. Before I tell you more about that, I want you to meet Sherry and Carlee.

SHERRY'S STORY

What I really enjoyed about meeting Carlee and Sherry was that these two concepts of being honest, and a daughter being able to see right through a mother, were written all over their story as mother and daughter. Sherry, if you were to meet her, seems to be a delightful mix of a sensitive-reflective capacity, and downright powerhouse of a woman; a rare combination to be found in such a beautifully put-together woman. To get to know her more, and set up for our interview, I asked her about her story of growing up, and how she became who she is today. Sherry described her childhood as rich with activities, sports and camping, where she was the "tomboy" who generally felt good about herself. The story becomes more complex when she describes going through puberty, and not getting her period until she was sixteen. This made her feel unlike the rest of her friends, who had had their first period long before. She started to mistrust her body and ask herself, "I wonder if it's ever going to happen." I found it interesting to note all of the things she said throughout this part of our interview, such as, "I was never a tiny girl," which implied so much more than what was actually said. If I read between the lines, this tells me that especially around puberty she was aware of how her body looked, compared to what society expected of girls her age. In spite of her awareness of size, and wondering about when she would develop like her friends, her appearance didn't seem to be something that defined her. She says that she dressed to suit her shape and size in a way that allowed her to feel good about her appearance.

When her husband was twenty-eight and Sherry was twenty-seven, her husband was diagnosed with cancer, and the priorities in the family shifted. The goal was to become and stay as healthy as possible, both individually, and as a family. She had three young children at home, one of whom was Carlee, and she says that she did her best during those years of her husband's recovery. I forgot to ask at the time what she meant by that, but rereading her interview I think it means she tried to keep her family alive, in all sense of the word, letting life stay as normal as possible, and making sure everyone had what they needed. It seemed, however, that it all caught up with her. She told me without shyness that at thirty she had a nervous breakdown. But as she started to speak about how difficult life was at that time, her voice dropped in a way that told me she was telling me something painful for her. She told me about the times she was immobilized by her anxiety, and how powerless she felt. Through the guidance and support of her doctor, she was put on a medication that ended up causing her to gain weight rapidly. This was hard for her, and posed a new kind of challenge as she worked hard to accept herself as she was: the new fragile sense of self, the weight gain, it all.

As with Anne, whom you met in the previous chapter, Sherry's mother never took time to educate her about women's bodies. She is certain that what her mother did and how she acted was enough to communicate to her healthy messages about bodies. She describes her mom eating healthy portions of healthy food, and playing tennis lots and encouraging Sherry to do the same. In fact, it was her grandfather who helped her, practically and emotionally, with the ins and outs of puberty. This made my jaw drop, thinking about my grandfather taking me to buy my first bra or tampons, instead of my mom. This seems, in my mind, like a sacred rite of passage between a mother and a daughter, a series of events in the initiation to womanhood by a woman. Sherry seemed ok with it, though; after all, it was what she knew. She did remember having closeness with her mom, although that has since changed. Her mom now, as she ages, has become much more emotionally dependent on Sherry, which she experiences as violating her boundaries. She can see that her mother is hurting, but doesn't want her mom to rely on her so much that she's totally dependent on Sherry emotionally. This struggle is so common to many daughters as their mothers age—how as women do we do for our mothers without it taking over our identities and priorities as an adult daughter? I can imagine that as women we will wrestle with that question differently depending on our relationships with our mother, our cultural background, our mother's needs and our abilities to meet them, and how many other siblings we have.

The closeness Sherry had with her mother early on is something that she wanted to recreate with her daughter Carlee. She said a few times while we were talking that she is curious about what Carlee said to me in our interview together. But she also wants to protect Carlee's space by saying, "I don't pry, it's not my place." That respectful curiosity was something I so admired in her, desiring to know her daughter more, but recognizing that her daughter's thoughts and feelings are her own. She is reflective, and talked about wanting to be close to Carlee in many ways, but also give her daughter space just to be herself. One of the ways she feels she has been honest with her daughter in a healthy way has been to speak honestly with Carlee, and her other children, about her own struggles. She did this in a way that told her children the truth about her life, but not in a way that would make her kids feel they needed to care for or parent her in return. She told me about letting her kids know about her struggles with anxiety in a way that was age-appropriate for them. She told me about letting her kids know about her own insecurities, and how she's managed them throughout her life. She told me that she's been honest with her kids about how not having a career has impacted her self-worth. At times, this made her feel like she didn't have much to offer in the world, and that she was *just* a "wife" or "mom." When we were talking about this, we joked about how people often ask each other "so what do you do?" when they meet for the first time, and how this reminded her, even recently, about her struggle with answering this question. She told all her kids (here comes the ladder) that she wanted them to follow their dreams in life, and aspire to more than just getting married, but to have a career that was all their own.

What I think you might particularly admire while listening to Sherry's story is how clearly she has been able to see the beauty in all of her struggles. About Carlee she says "she's very close to her dad. ... One of the benefits of me being sick was that my husband pitched in with the children, and all of my kids have a really good relationship with their dad. They've gone traveling with him, 'cause I couldn't travel, it just gave me anxiety. ... I've become a better person for it, I'm much more accepting, I'm much more aware." What is particularly unique about this part of her story is how Sherry describes the healthy relationships which blossomed out of her years of illness: her children and their dad, and her relationship with herself. She has, no doubt communicated this concept of personal-growth-through-challenge idea to her kids, and reminded them that in spite of our struggles and pain, we can learn to accept ourselves even more, and grow.

Because of this unique part of their story as mother and daughter, I asked Sherry exactly what she told Carlee about her struggles with anxiety. I wanted to know how she was able to be honest with her daughter in a way that didn't make Carlee feel responsible for her mom's anxiety, but could help Carlee learn from her mom instead. She probably had lots of questions too, about why her dad was taking her on trips and her mom wasn't coming. And, like many of the clients I see whose children see them taking medication, ask, "Mommy, why are you taking those pills? Will I have to take them when I grow up like you?" She says that unlike my struggle, where I am worried about passing on body-shame and disordered eating to my future daughter, she was worried about passing on anxiety to hers. She said, "Talk to me about anxiety, I could tell you a whole lot … because that's my experience. Yours is food and eating. Mine has been anxiety. I could answer those questions for you for days. … I've got a [good idea] about what I've told my girls, because this is my reality." She says she remembered vividly telling them about anxiety, in general, and what you could do about it if you had it. She says she made a point of asking her kids about their own worries, and letting them know that she always wanted them to tell her about their feelings and fears. It sounded like she was nowhere near having them sit down and pretend they were her therapists, and talk endlessly to them for hours about her own problems. But, she did say things like "this is what Mom is going through" and "if you have problems like this, here's what you can do about it." In short, "You're not crazy, and you're not alone." She gave them a mental "map" of how to get back to feeling good, when they were lost in feeling overwhelmed and anxious.

Because anxiety had been such a struggle for her, she says that she doesn't have any memory of what she told Carlee about weight and body image. Instead, she talked more about healthy living and dealing with anxiety. I said to Sherry, "Tell me more about what you explicitly communicated to Carlee about your own body," and she replied decisively, "Nothing." Shocked, especially since she had been so vocal about so many other things, I said to her, probably insensitively, "You can't remember what you might have said?" and again she said, "NOPE, no." She had the same answer when I asked her more similar questions related to what she might have communicated without knowing it. Where this gets interesting is when we start to put together the pieces about how differently her mother remembers the story than Carlee does. I'll get to that after I introduce you to Carlee.

CARLEE'S STORY

I have actually known Carlee, at a distance, for a few years. When I got in contact with her for the interview, she reminded me that we had met several years ago on campus while doing our undergraduate degrees at the same university. Carlee is powerful in a way that might make some people feel shy: she has a firm, strong voice, radiant smile, and a glimmer in her eyes that makes you think she has probably pulled a few good pranks in her lifetime. When she's talking to you, she'll unapologetically stare you dead in the eye. She is tough, you can tell, and has the heart of a fighter.

Carlee describes having felt powerful from a young age, and does still now—especially when she plays hockey. And what is so intriguing about her is that she is shamelessly herself. She says that her mom has always focused on who she was as a person, not on her weight. About her mom, she says "she was just letting me be me." When Carlee tells me the story of being in her body, she says "my body has always been the same to me, I've always had hips, I've never been like that size 2 really thin, not even as a child." She mentioned, like most other women, that puberty meant a change in how her body looked and felt, but there was something so beautiful and unique about her interpretation of that. She says, "I knew I'd get hips, my mom has hips. I thought, 'Yes, I was meant to have children,' like, I've always wanted to have children, so I find that it's powerful thing that I have hips, that I have curves. It's great."

In the moment, hearing her say that, I remember thinking, "Wow, who says that?" I feel the same way now. Carlee has been able to embrace some of the things that make us most womanly, and consequently in our society most ashamed. Instead of shaming her body for becoming more feminine, more mature, she connected with the sacred power of the feminine form. When I asked her about if she's ever felt shame about her body, she confidently replied that she's always felt this way about her body. I probed more when she told me about times when she was younger and she wanted to wear shorts over her bathing suit at the beach. But, she said this to indicate that it might have looked to those on the outside like she was ashamed or insecure, but she felt it was a protective modesty. It was her way of taking care of herself, not putting on display for everyone else the parts of her that were most intimate. She often chooses to dress out of respect for herself, to honor how sacred she believes she and her body are, together.

She doesn't recall having shamed herself, but she did tell me that there have been moments when she's questioned her security in herself when noticing she had some cellulite. She told me, however, that the more she thought about it, she came to the conclusion that if anyone else shamed her because of how her thighs looked, or found cellulite to be a barrier to loving her, that they would not be worth her time. When she thinks about meeting someone, and falling in love, she says, "If I meet someone, and they don't want to be with me because I have cellulite on my legs, they're not worth it. No! And, if I'm friends with anyone who's like, 'Oh did you see her legs?' like, it's absurd, I am who I am, I love my body." She reminded me when she said this that even people who completely love their bodies doubt themselves sometimes, and see themselves through the lens that culture gives us as women. What's different about Carlee is that she can respond critically to these messages and remind herself that she is so much more than if she has cellulite or not, and that if her legs look a certain way or not is not what defines her relationship with herself.

She talks about pushing her mom's buttons, and being able to do that now as an adult because of the strength of their relationships and because she believes her mom can handle it; in other words, they are safe with each other, and in themselves. Carlee says that she's always felt safe to challenge her mother's opinions, and speak up if she didn't like something. That powerful bond seemed to be there in ways from the beginning, but came especially as Sherry reinforced to Carlee over time that she didn't have to be perfect, and that she was beautiful and wonderful just as she was. She remembers always feeling secure in her mother's love, and never worrying that her mom, or dad, would stop loving her, ever.

We spoke a little bit more about this, and Carlee remembers on countless occasions her mom telling Carlee the truth about herself. She says of her mom, "She would tell me I was beautiful. … It wasn't like every day, but you know … I think she just built me up more through the characteristics that I had." What interested me about this statement was how Sherry had been vocal about telling Carlee that she was beautiful. But, the way Sherry told Carlee about her beauty had more to it than just her looks; she built up Carlee's character and told her that she was good at things, and kind, and smart, and powerful. After she mentioned this, we discussed the trickiness of telling your daughter who she is, and how great she looks, but not in such a way that overemphasizes her appearance. I said back to her, "I imagine if she had told you that you looked beautiful every day, except on days you didn't do your hair, then all of a sudden you're learning implicitly that good hair equals beautiful," and consequently, bad hair means not beautiful. And the games begin.

It seems like it could be so tricky, trying to figure out how to tell your daughter who she is, and be honest and firm, while also not just focusing on one aspect of who she is. Because, when you're telling her who she is, you *do* need to address her looks and body. That is one important part of her, but it's not all she is: she is a heart, a brain, a friend, a learner, a creator, and probably many more things. As I'm writing this, I'm thinking back to the bank account analogy I used in the previous chapter to emphasize how small things matter, especially over a lifetime. Now think about it like this: you have a few different accounts, and some of those accounts you use all the time. There are other accounts, like savings or investment accounts, that you rarely touch, and only to make big withdrawals or deposits every so often. It takes a little bit of organizing, but you are able to keep track of which accounts you need to put more money into, and when. Imagine, for a moment, the horribly simplistic idea that your daughter is a set of bank accounts, and that all the parts of who she is are represented in separate accounts. The "appearance-body" account gets a lot of withdrawals because every day she is hearing lies about herself from the media, and culture, and probably people around her. So, that is going to need more deposits from you. But, there are other accounts that matter too, like her creativity, independence, and compassion accounts. Those need some attention, and can't be ignored.

In fact, I imagine that one of the most difficult parts of all this is figuring out which "accounts" your daughter needs you to "fill up"—because she probably needs to hear things from you sometimes that you never knew she struggled with. Maybe she's a good student and you have no idea she's worried about grades and being "good enough," and because she's not telling you it's hard for you to know that she needs that from you.

Sherry probably had no idea how Carlee would grow up to reflect on what she said or did. But when I asked her about it, Carlee said, "She wasn't telling me who I had to be … she was just letting me be me, and if I wanted to wear baggy shorts, baggy T-shirts, play football or whatever— I'm very thankful that she focused on who I was as a person, and not on the body, my body, or like the image, or what I looked like physically. I think that was huge."

A NOTE ON INCONSISTENCIES

As I mentioned at the start of the chapter, daughters are good at picking up the inconsistencies in the stories. Both Carlee and Sherry, in their separate interviews, told me about a time when Carlee was a young and how her mother had paid her to grow her hair out. Instead, she chose to keep it short because she liked it that way. In this story, both mother and daughter were able to see after many years how the messages were inconsistent with the rest of what Sherry told and showed Carlee. Her mother had both said to her, "I think you're perfect just as you are," and then tried to put on Carlee her preferences for a feminine "girly-girl." Carlee noticed the inconsistency because it "stuck out"—this incident was an outlier. Because her mom normally fought for her freedom, strength, and independence, Carlee could resist her mom's wish for her to have long hair, and this seemed easier to roll off her back.

Carlee also remembers that on a number of occasions her mother made comments about being dissatisfied with how she feels about her own looks. She says that her mom has told her daughter that she wants to be more active, and that she has said a number of times, "If I'm thin when I die, I'd like to be buried in my bikini." Sherry also said things while shopping with her daughter, like, "I don't ever want to have to go to a plus-sized store." These messages about her own body communicated to Carlee that there was an inconsistency between how she saw herself, and how she saw her daughter. Daughters notice these kinds of things, when mothers say or do things differently for or to their daughters than for themselves. While this is healthier than if moms were to figuratively beat their daughters up, as they beat themselves up in their own heads, their girls can't help but start to wonder and ask themselves questions about growing up.

When I asked Sherry about some of these things, as I wrote earlier, she recalled having always been more preoccupied with telling her daughter the truth about worries, anxiety, and feelings, than bodies and weight. And, that's probably how these messages go through. She wasn't intentionally trying to say things about herself that didn't match what she said about her daughter. They probably just slipped out, without her knowing her daughter would remember them, and then talk about them in an interview years later.

In this example, I saw something I encounter a lot when working with moms: they desperately want their children to experience freedom and independence, but this is particularly difficult if they want something different than what their mothers want. Because moms want the best for their daughters, they might confuse what is best for them, or what they have believed is the best, with what their daughter might need. It might be interesting to think about some of the things that your mother said or did through her eyes, how what she wanted for herself translated to what she wanted for you. If you're a mother, think of yourself in Sherry's shoes— what might your preferences and expectations be for your daughter? Is it possible that those are things that *you* want *for* her, but might not be what she wants for her?

ABUSE AND SHAME

As a therapist, I find it hard to write about this, without also addressing the exceptions: abuse of any kind is never a good thing. If you received that at the hand of your mother (or anyone else, ever), I am so sorry that happened to you. You did not deserve it. And if as a mother you are engaging in abuse of your daughter, or anyone for that matter, especially because you believe it is good for them, I urge you to find someone to speak to about this, and help you find more effective and healthy ways to have relationships. The other exceptions are when you as a parent know that something is good for your child, but she doesn't want it, such as helping your daughter take the medication she badly needs for an infection, going to school, or brushing her teeth. So, when thinking about what we want for others, it is important to distinguish between preferences for how they act based on gender (and all the rules we have always believed about "what good girls do") and what is essential for their well-being and health.

Although it may not be as immediately obvious to point out as some forms of abuse, using shame to parent can be effective, but insidious, nefarious, and extremely destructive to the person on the receiving end. One theory about shame feelings is that they arise to help us conform with societal or cultural expectations—to help us secure a feeling of belonging, or at least prevent us from feeling the pain of being an outsider. It wasn't long ago that using shame to parent was a popular strategy to change a child's behavior. Parenting with shame happens when we use the threat of disconnection and conditional love to try and force a person to change something. Maybe it was something used in your home growing up to get you to pick your clothes or toys off the floor, or dress or act a certain way in public. Maybe it's literally been the voice of someone in your family saying to you "you will never be loved if you keep eating that much dessert." And, shame works. It feels so awful that we usually want to change the behavior to make the feeling go away. But it generally sticks around longer than we thought it would, or than the person who shamed us knew it could. It can embed itself in our identity deeply, generalizing from the thing we weren't "supposed to do" to who we are, leaving us feeling unlovable and unworthy of acceptance or belonging. If you were shamed a lot, or at all, growing up, it's likely you still remember it. These are memories that are often hard to forget, shaping our behaviors, styles of interaction, or beliefs about ourselves.

WHAT HAPPENED IN THE MOTHERS AND DAUGHTERS?

There was a theme among all the young healthy women: their mothers did an awesome job, and some negative body-dissatisfied comments snuck through. And, the daughters took note of and recalled these exceptions, because they were by and large the exceptions. This, in the grand scheme of things, is also really unique: the daughters felt like their mothers were so consistent and affirming in how they spoke to them about their beauty that when anything else or different was said, they were able to pick it out right away. This ability to think critically, and see the discrepancy in their mothers' stories, is probably in part why they were able to be so healthy and love themselves. They were able to think about messages, instead of just blindly accepting them to be true. I'll talk more about that in a later chapter, as it relates to culture and the media.

Although up to now I've mostly told you about mothers telling the truth about themselves to their daughter, an equally important job is to always tell your daughter the truth about who she is. And, you need to keep telling her those truths about herself even if she wears the "I'm-too-cool-to-acknowledge-I-feel-good-when-you-say-that" mask. In the world, there are a lot of messages quite readily circulated about who she is which aren't a reflection of her true worth, value, and identity. She needs to hear the truth from you—not just about your own story, but also about hers. I think we can expand this to the greater community of women: we could listen more to each other, and tell each other when we see their greatness, passion, determination and beauty. And, when they are hurting, we can tell them, and show them the truth—that they are not alone.

I asked every one of the healthy, self-loving daughters about what they would want to say on this subject to their daughters or future daughters one day. And almost all of them mentioned some kind of "truth telling": they wanted their daughters to know the truth about how they learned to love themselves as they are. They all believed that if their daughters knew the truths about their mothers' struggles, instead of harming their future daughters, it would help them if they ever found themselves in the same spot. This is exactly what Sherry did for Carlee, because of her struggle with anxiety. Kelsey, whom you met in the previous chapter, said, "I'd want to be honest with her and say … 'it was a journey, and it was a process.' … You do have your times where you look at yourself and it's difficult for yourself, but you can overcome them and work through them, and you can receive healing in those areas to teach her to have compassion for herself in the times where she my look in the mirror and say "oh I'm ugly." Like Carlee, Kelsey saw in her own mom the discrepancies between how she saw herself and what she said to her daughter. And instead of hiding it, the daughters all felt like speaking truth about the world, and their stories, was the best way to protect their daughters.

When I got on the phone with Sherry for the first time to ask her if I could interview her, I told her a little bit about why I wanted to interview her along with other women and their mothers. I told her that for my own life, I'm not going to be satisfied if I see a problem and don't do something about it. I told her that I have committed my life to helping people who are hurt, and in particular people who have been hurt in areas that I've been hurt. She said that when I said this, when I was honest and vulnerable about my story, and told her my hopes, she acknowledged, "I let my guard down." Then she laughed and said, "You ask my girls, or you ask my husband, I don't sit down with a complete stranger and talk, it's not who I am." When I reread this part of the transcript from the interview that I had with Sherry, I felt a shiver run down my body. I didn't know why at first, so I mulled it over in my mind for a few days. Just as I sat down to finish this chapter I finally understood why her story impacted me so much;

she was thinking about you—reading this, right now. She was thinking about how much more important it was in that moment to be honest, than to hide under the fear of what could happen if she took her mask off. She did this so she could help us all. Sherry's struggle with anxiety is not something she advertises to everyone, which may not be obvious based on how candidly she spoke to me. Until the interview, I was a stranger to her. She could have easily worn a mask with me and told me that her life had been perfect, and would continue to be perfect, without exception. Or she could have easily not done the interview at all. Instead, what she did was tell me the truth about her life, because she ultimately knew that sharing her honest story with me would help me get this book to you, and that you might learn something from her. She said, "In my experience in life there is pain, and hurt, and anxiety, and it's not fun to go through, but you can, after you've walked through all the fuzz and the garbage, you can see good. Sometimes right in the middle of it, you can't."

Telling the truth about our lives, to the right people, at the right time, can make all the difference. This is not only true for us among women, as fellow travelers, but also among generations of women. It is important for those who have gone before us to tell us what they've been through so that we can learn from them, or realize we're not alone. We need each other as women, and that is especially true of mothers and daughters. Daughters cannot be their mothers' therapists. But, your daughter does need to hear from you about what you learned in your struggles, so that she may benefit from your mistakes and suffering. A friend of mine, who is also a therapist, used the term with me the other day: "speaking from scars and not from wounds." In this she's saying that there is a difference between going to our children with gaping, open emotional wounds that they are not capable of or responsible for fixing, and knowing when we've walked through something that has been painful and has shaped us in some way that we can talk about it with them from a place of knowing that it's over, and we got through it.

It is easy for many of us as women to joke about the fear of becoming our mothers. For some of us, who were truly and deeply hurt by them, that could be a very real fear. For others of us, it is something that feels uncomfortable, but mostly a hilarious inevitability. I think I'm in the latter category. Amidst the pain we have had in our relationship, and times when seeing the world differently has made it hard for us to understand each other, or has even made us hurt each other, I see the beauty, strength, and resilience in my mother. I'd like to be different than who she is, but mostly because I want to be *me*. I'm not afraid anymore of being like her. But I want to be the fullest version of who I am, and I imagine that that will make us both similar and different in many ways. I can feel peace with that, as well as a fear that has shifted towards having a daughter. I'm afraid I will hurt her, I'm afraid she will hurt like I hurt when I was growing up. I'm afraid that I will not understand her, or know how to give her what she needs. Maybe that is a projection of the unresolved hurts I have in my relationship with my mom—not wanting to recreate the fragments in my relationship with a daughter that I have so readily felt between my mother and me. Or maybe it's because I feel the weight of even the potential of a new and precious life: wanting to give a sacred life everything she deserves.

If one day I have a daughter, I hope I can sit her down and tell her the truth about myself. I'll probably need to apologize and say something about how I am doing my best, and will always want to and try to do better. I know already there will have to be many times of saying "sorry" and "please forgive me." I know that I will also want to tell her the truth about herself, and help her learn that being a woman doesn't mean we have to be perfect. And, that so much healing can happen in ourselves and for others when we can tell each other what we've learned and how to get through it. I hope I'll be able to tell her then that I love myself more than ever before, that that hasn't always been the case, but that our journeys in life do not have to be perfect to be magnificent and victorious.

REFLECTION QUESTIONS

- What were the ways in which your body was talked about, and not talked about?
- What might be some of the ways that you act and speak that contradict the other?
- What did your mother do and say about her body, and your body? Were those messages consistent?
- If you were to have a daughter one day, what would you want to be able to tell her about your life, about who you are and what shaped you?
- What do you wish you could go back and tell your younger self about growing up?

▶ If you have a daughter…
- What are the ways that you encourage your daughter?
- What have you left out when you're encouraging her?
- Who are the people in your life who you might need to take your mask off with? How do you know that you're ready, that they're ready?
- What kind of lessons have you learned through your struggles that you could tell your daughter?
- What's one way, today, that you could tell her the truth about who she is? ("You're so special to me, you are 'enough' as you are, you're not alone in this world, you are beautiful just as you are, being beautiful is not the most important thing about you, you are so …")
- What are your preferences, and how might those be different than the essentials—either for your daughter or for yourself? Where did these preferences come from?

FOUR

SAFETY AND AFFIRMATION: MORE THAN ENOUGH LOVE

"How bold one gets when one is sure of being loved."

–FREUD

There is a young woman I've been working with in therapy for almost two years now. She called me originally because she had started to think about ending her life in a way that felt so real it scared her. She was a new mom with a daughter who was only six months old. I asked her the usual questions I ask a new client so I could get to know her, and in the process she could get to know me. Right away I started to notice a few things. She was highly accomplished, well-educated, and successful at her work, and had one of the most profound issues of self-worth that I have ever seen.

When she was growing up her family ran a business. From a very early age she was given lots of opportunities to help out. Even chores that she did for allowance money were related to tasks that needed to be done for the business. As she started high school, it was assumed that she would be working at the business after school each day and on weekends, and some of the most awful fights she had with her mother were when she

46

announced she was going to try and get a job running summer camps at the local community center. She remembers her mom telling her one spring afternoon, when she was in ninth grade, that her duty as a member of the family was to support the family business. And as a result, she wasn't going to be able to run the summer camp. Her mom had implied this on several occasions, but actually said it during one of those fights: she was not going to be valued or belong in the family unless she could prove to them that she was lightening the burden of the business.

Having done such work from an early age, and then growing up with business conversation and language around the dinner table, she began to excel in certain courses in high school. When she graduated, she started in a degree program at a university so she could work towards filling in for her dad when he wanted to retire. She graduated with honors, and continued on in school for a few more years to finish a certificate that she needed to be licensed at the highest level in her field.

I remember sitting across from her in our first session, listening intently, but plagued by the questions of who she really was. I was learning all about her, but was sitting there yearning to know who she was underneath the obvious achievements. I remember seeing all of the external accomplishments, the lovely appearance, the well-spoken woman sitting in front of me, and still wondering if I was just seeing a version of her that her mother and father had created, or if I was seeing who she really was.

So I asked her, "If you could do anything else in the world for work, besides what you're doing, what would you do"? She sat, very still, without speaking a word, for almost five minutes, then said, "I'd do what I'm doing for another company." I thought, for sure, she had misunderstood my question. I had wanted to know if she got to explore any other facet of life, or work, what would that be. I asked again, and tried to clarify the question, and she said very quietly after a few moments, "I don't know, this is all I've ever done." As she said this, a few tears rolled gently down her face.

As we continued our work together, we were able to figure out that she had never really been allowed to be herself. She always saw herself, and I believe she was directly told and shown this repeatedly, that she was only valuable in the family if she did something to help the business, but for no other reason did she have worth. This created a fierce lack of self-worth, and made her feel like she was always running a race to prove to others that she was good enough. Unless she came in first, she was a failure. But now, sitting in my office with a brand new baby girl, she was just so tired of running.

I can imagine that having a daughter is hard, especially for the experienced and wise mother seeing her making choices you disagree with. I'm not talking about if she is going to do drugs or get a neck tattoo for her thirteenth birthday; those are choices that as her mother you're encouraged to disagree with and let her know you're the parent. But I'm talking about when she makes choices to start dressing like a tomboy when you think that looking feminine in pink is the way to go. Or, if she decides she wants to cut her hair short, or dye it a certain color, that doesn't fit the image you have for your family. Or, you come from a family of cheerleaders, and she wants to learn to play guitar and join a garage band. I can imagine that it's hard when she starts to become her own person, and that is different than who you are, or who you wanted her to become. I don't think it's wrong to want things for her, but I do believe that it's important to remember that what you want for her isn't necessarily who she is. And what you want may say more about what's important for you than what's best for her.

What we all need and deserve is to know, right from the beginning, that no matter who we are, we are loved and lovable. If you have a daughter now or one day, what's most important is that she knows that no matter who she is, no matter what she does, you will love her. And, that you will never stop loving her. In order to do this, you will have to separate her behavior from her worth. This means that when her behavior is bad, or she makes bad decisions, that you can point them out and support her

KRENUS, AU

All the devils are h

31010002971119

to change them, but that she never feels like your love will ever get taken away. She needs to know that you love her, and that she doesn't have to earn it. We all need to learn how to do this. The things we do cannot be the way that we determine if we're valuable or lovable. Feeling like our worth and value is conditional upon what we do, how well we perform, and what others think about us, can be destructive to our identity, our mental health, our relationships. And it can create a life where we are running, proving, and searching to get or keep the interest of others, without ever really knowing who we are. This is something that the young woman I was telling you about never knew; she truly believed that she was only loved or lovable if she did things for her parents to help the business. Instead of existing in the world with confidence and courage, her feelings and choices were governed by shame, insecurity, lack of self-worth, and fear.

ATTACHMENT

There is actually research showing that how loved and secure a daughter feels in her relationship with her mother can actually predict if she's more likely to have issues with her body or eating, or not. The word we use to describe the relationship she has with you is called "attachment." Psychologists and researchers have been able to categorize attachment into a few different "styles" or patterns; just think of them as categories of relationship. Part of what happens when people have healthy attachment (think an optimal relationship with their primary caregivers growing up) is that they generally feel ok about themselves, and safe in the world. They know they belong, and are lovable. They are more likely to grow up to have a relationship with a partner that is based on mutual trust, connection, and relational-emotional-physical safety. When people have unhealthy attachment style (really difficult, frightening, cold/distant, abusive, inconsistent or nonexistent relationship with their primary caregiver) they tend to have a hard time feeling ok with themselves, handling painful or powerful emotions, and believing they're safe, or won't be abandoned. They are more likely to grow up to be distant, anxious, and/or insecure in their romantic relationship, or choose people who replicate these unhealthy patterns from growing up. Children actually need to be shown, relentlessly, that you love them, won't leave them, and that you will keep them safe. It's pretty hard for them to believe that those things are true unless you prove to them that they're true by what you do.

We all want to belong and know that we're good enough. As girls and as women, we're told from the moment we're born that belonging and good "enoughness" comes from how we look. We are told as women that we need to be beautiful, and if we're beautiful, or thin, or sexy, or pretty, that we're desirable, and "good enough." For women in our culture (and sadly, increasingly for boys and young men), a lot of our worth comes down to how we look. So just imagine for a second that a young girl has never learned that she is "enough as she is," that she is unique, and has the right to make choices about how she wants to be in the world. And she goes through high school and all of a sudden she notices that all the thin girls get more attention from the boys. When she loses weight herself, she notices that other people like her, tell her she's pretty, and she starts to feel really good about herself. Because, for the first time in her life, she's felt accepted and seen, a part of her gets caught up in it all because she finally feels like she has worth for the first time.

This is a fairly simplistic explanation of the relationship between attachment and body image, or disordered eating, but I wanted to try and help you see the links. Women and girls in our world are told over and over again that they get their worth through looking a certain way. And unless she learns otherwise, this is going to be the case. One study published in 2012[4] demonstrated the links between a young woman's attachment style with her mother and if she was dissatisfied with her body. What's most interesting about this study was that young women who were considered to have an anxious attachment style (thought highly of others, low of themselves, and were worried about being abandoned) were more likely to idealize and internalize the images of thin women in the media, and feel poorly about themselves. These research findings are not new, or the first to say this kind of thing, with lots of other recent studies showing the same results.[5]

If you're a mom, and in particular if you're a mom who has a daughter who struggles with her body image and weight in some way, this is not meant to make you feel blame or shame, but instead to remind you just how important you are. She needs you, maybe even more than anyone else. And she doesn't need you to be perfect, but she needs you to be there in whatever ways you can. She needs to know that you love her, that you're there for her, and that even if she's annoying and frustrating and moody that you will never stop loving her. She needs to know that you will never abandon her, physically or emotionally.

The pattern of attachment that we learned early on is something that can show up in our close relationships with others (or can get in the way of us forming close relationships with others), especially with romantic partners. Sometimes as adults we are drawn to people with whom we can replicate our early attachment patterns. Even if a relationship isn't healthy, it might feel comfortable—it might be that with that person we can fit into an old relational pattern or groove. What is important to know is that as adults, and especially in romantic relationships, our partners have a similar role in speaking into our lives, as do parents when we're a child growing up. The relationship links we have with people other than our mothers shape us too; what they say counts. If you're in a romantic relationship, have been in the past, or hope to be in the future, think about what your partner has said about your body and your appearance, and how that made you feel about yourself. And think about what you have said about your partner's body and appearance, and how it may have made them feel. Maybe we are so used to hearing something hurtful that we don't even realize how hurtful it is. Or, out of a place of hurt we say hurtful things back to our partner. To help us understand what might be healthy or unhealthy to hear or say, try thinking about it this way: if you or your partner say things to each other (about bodies and appearance) that you would never dream of saying to your child, then that's probably a good indication that they are hurtful or damaging things. It can be worth asking why you have allowed someone so close and important to you to say such hurtful things that you would never allow a person to say to someone else you care about. It can also be worth asking—if we're used to hurting or saying mean things to the people who are closest to us—what that's about for us, and where we learned to do that. The attachment relationships that we have shape how we feel about ourselves. It's also possible that we can be drawn to relationships which confirm how we already feel about ourselves. And, how we feel about ourselves affects not just our overall feelings towards our self (self-esteem), but our body image, and how we take up space and move through the world. After all, both self-esteem and attachment relationships do not exist in a vacuum, and are related to all parts of us, including our bodies. So, hurt in one area of our life can create or metastasize into hurt in another part of our life. Or if we feel loved exactly as we are by our partner, and our partner expresses that to us in a variety of ways, that will influence our feelings about and in our bodies, as it does all parts of ourselves. Healing in one part of our life can lead to healing in another area of our life. Freedom in one area can bleed into freedom in another area. They are all connected.*

BARBARA'S STORY

When thinking about how this chapter started—the story of a young woman who felt she had to be something or do something to feel loved or valuable—it may not be surprising that the moms in this study did something different for their daughters. They let them be themselves, and even if this was "weird to them," they loved their daughters anyway. A good example of this is in the story of Barbara, and her daughter Becky. Barbara is an accomplished mother of two. She has lived on different

---

* This is not to say that we should look to our partners exclusively to affirm our satisfaction with our appearance. But if someone we love shows and tells us that they love us no matter what, exactly as we are, that can help create or add to a storehouse of self-compassion that reminds us that our appearance isn't the only thing that's important about us.

continents, and after getting her PhD moved back to her home country to teach music at a local college. I had the chance to interview her in her office—full of books and sheet music. When I walked in, she was sitting behind a big desk, the semester had just ended, and she was in the midst of marking papers.

When Barbara talked about her body throughout her interview, she did so almost exclusively through comparison, particularly to her sister, who she considers to be more thin and gorgeous than herself. It seemed that the comparison between them started from a young age; when they were younger, her sister would point out Barbara's weight and she remembers feeling uncomfortable with her body even then. When I asked her to tell me more about that discomfort, and some of her early memories of feeling shame about her body, she told me a story about when her father picked her up and shook her as a child, calling her "as heavy as a sack of potatoes." When she said this she laughed, but she also looked sad, like she could almost remember how hurt that made her feel. She acknowledged the contradiction of those two, the laughing and the hurt saying that she was shocked that she remembered that seemingly insignificant comment, but it must have really affected her in some way, if, almost 50 years later, she could still remember it. She remembered how secretive she felt she had to be about getting her period for the first time. Acknowledging the social differences between then and now she says, "Nowadays, the guys and girls in high school, they talk about it, but it sure wasn't that way then."

Puberty was difficult for Barbara, as for most of the other women in this book, as it is for most of us. Around the time of her first period, she describes that a deep rift began to grow between her and her body. Inheriting the "family hips" made it hard to buy clothes and "camouflage" parts of herself she didn't like. She told me about gaining weight when she was pregnant, and how she felt she could allow herself to do so during that special part of her life. I have heard this from lots of women: the role of pregnancy is a socially sanctioned way for women to gain weight without shame. Like other women, she accepted her body as it was changing—unlike how it is considered by most women normally, the weight gain of pregnancy was a good thing.

Barbara seems to have a complicated relationship with her body where she is constantly balancing between staying healthy and not eating too much. Like Sherry and Anne, Barbara has found menopause to be a difficult transition, like a second puberty of sorts, where she's had to get to know a body which, again, is feeling strange and unfamiliar. But when I asked her to finish the sentence "my body is," she said without too much thought "my body is functional, everything works, and I'm thankful for that." I got the sense while listening to Barbara that she thinks of her body as a machine; her body is important, something which needs to be cared for, but it really is just something that carries her "self" around. Within her there appears to be a self-acceptance laced through her view of her body as well, and she treats her body/machine well because she believes it is a gift from God, and it's her responsibility to care for it, whether she likes it or not.

When Barbara told me about her mother, and their relationship, there were some things we both picked up on that she probably learned from her. She said her mother was always telling her about what a good woman dressed and looked like, and that there were certain ways of being a woman that were not appropriate: wearing skirts that were too short, or showing too much skin. Her mother, however, didn't actually say much about bodies. She said about this lack of conversation, "The culture of that generation ... the European culture, you really didn't talk much about things, so I can't really remember her saying really much of anything." Although her mom was relatively silent about her own body, and her daughters' bodies, Barbara always remembers feeling very safe, cared for, and loved by her mother. When her older sister would make comments about Barbara's weight, her mom would defend Barbara. She recalls her mother "never" said anything negative about anyone, and that she was an amazing friend who supported people and loved them no matter what they looked like. If she did say something at all about a person's weight, Barbara remembers that this was only ever to express concern for their health and well-being. Although she's not perfectly thrilled with how she looks, or how her aging body is functioning, I thought she finished the sentence "women's bodies are" so beautifully. She said "women's bodies are varied. There are so many beautiful women, but it really has nothing to do with their size or their shape; there is so much variety and it can all be beautiful." I want to believe this, I want us all to believe this, and even though Barbara said it, I was left wondering if she was able to believe this for herself.

When I asked her about her relationship with her daughter Becky, she told me about how she made a conscious effort to have more dialogue about life, and bodies, and womanhood with her daughter than her mother had with her. When she was young, Becky asked her mother all the time about her birth story, and marriage: the simple curiosity of a young girl wanting to get to know her mother, and herself. But, when their family moved back to North America after having lived abroad for a number of years, she remembers that Becky stopped talking to her and that it made her sad to feel that distance between herself and her daughter. She had been longing to be close to Becky as she grew up, and after they moved, around the time that Becky was thirteen, it all changed. Thinking back about that, Barbara's longing for closeness with her daughter was apparent: "I wish when she was a teenager that we could have talked more openly about things."

Like her mother, Barbara is concerned with Becky being a good woman, and looking "right," and she remembers being confused that Becky had no interest in wearing makeup, and often wanted to push that on her—to show her how to do her hair properly, or dress up fancy. But, careful to note that Becky is a natural beauty and "doesn't need makeup," Barbara was able to let go that how her daughter chose to dress and look was her own choice, and that she needed to be herself in the world, not a carbon copy of her mother. I was really interested in that part of their story—unlike so many of the other stories where the mothers were relatively silent, Barbara was really desiring to be open and close with her daughter and it was Becky who chose to pull away. I can imagine it would have been so easy for so many moms to feel hurt and bitter, and with resentment act in a way that communicates "if you don't want to be close to me, then I don't want to be close to you." What Barbara did, instead, was to try and stay engaged, to be present and in-tune with her daughter. She "warned" Becky about getting the big maternal hips that the other women in her family got, and reminded her that that was ok. She says she even was watching and waiting for Becky to get her period, and spoke to her a lot about it before she even got it for the first time. Like a lot of teenage girls, Becky got squeamish and said things like "oh, Mom, do we have to talk about this?" and Barbara stayed firm, but gentle, reminding Becky that she could talk to her about anything, and that she was young once too. She told me, "I wanted her to know that she could come to me at any time, if she had a concern about something, or if she was, you know, didn't know how to do something or whatever." I really admired that about how Barbara parented Becky—she didn't demand that Becky be close to her in order to try and be close back. And, she didn't wait until Becky asked about things, to tell her about the important stuff in life about being a woman.

COMPARISON

When Barbara talks about her daughter now, she describes a strong, creative, hard-working young woman. She is incredibly proud of who Becky is. Although Barbara didn't mention this in our interview, I wonder if she ever did compare herself to Becky, as she compared herself to her sister. Or, if she compared her relationship with her mom to her relationship with Becky. I wonder how Barbara learned to deal with the feelings she had when Becky was a teenager and didn't seem interested in building a relationship. Although comparison can pit us against each other as women, it can be one of the only ways we learn how to measure ourselves, our worth, our beauty, if we know that we're "making" it or not. If we're not measuring ourselves against a standard, a desired or ideal something or someone, how do we know if we are good enough? It's a logic most of us buy into as women, because deciding to not compare might only happen when we are willing to believe that, especially when it comes to looks, we are all different and ok just as we are. This means finding a new way of thinking about ourselves, and the people around us. And, for most of us, we're not ready. I believe that we all want to know that we're enough, but might not know how to hold that as true about ourselves unless we can prove it to ourselves by being more [insert your desired trait or appearance here] than someone else. The downfall of comparison is that when it comes to the "ideal," there will almost always be someone who is closer to it. So even if we're more thin/beautiful/funny/smart than someone else, we'll always have a reason to beat ourselves up about not being enough of those things either. Even for the people who actually manage to approximate the appearance ideal, when that is the way that they have earned their "enoughness," then they are trapped in the game of needing to maintain that ideal so they don't lose their "enoughness" to someone who is even more ideal. What if we quit the game? What if each of us were already enough, and gaining weight, losing weight, stretch marks, grey hair, wrinkles, cellulite, weren't things we were afraid of or had power over us? But were things, kind of like eye color, that maybe we noticed, but learned to work with, accept, and even enjoy because they were unique about us? What if these things in others, instead of being the ruler we used to measure ourselves against to feel bad or good about how we looked, were just things about other people that we noticed, but that was it? What if when we saw other people, or ourselves in the mirror, we saw a real three-dimensional human with hopes, wounds, losses, talents, and quirks that were unique, instead of a person we reduced to a series of physical characteristics? Comparison forces us to push each other away, seeing the differences, instead of joining together or seeing the beauty, the strengths, the common humanity. You can start singing "kum-ba-ya" now: I want that for all of us as women. Instead of objectifying ourselves and other women and then being cruel about what we see, being people who know that we are good enough just as we are, so that we can love other people into helping them believe that about themselves too. If we decide to quit the game of comparison-to-prove-worth, we can liberate each other and ourselves from a flattened, cruel, and shallow existence which really only serves to reduce us as humans to a few physical qualities, when we are so much more.

BECKY'S STORY

In spite of the two of them being very different people, Becky's interview—as with many other parts of who she is—reminded me a lot of her mother. We spoke about the same stories, the same fights and challenges, and the same "family hips" that came up in the interview with her mother. Like some of the other young women you're reading about, Becky referred to herself as a "tomboy." Because Becky grew up away from North America and the influences of Western media, she told me about a childhood where she played sports with her friends. But puberty was hard for her. She recalls, "I started developing hips, and that really threw me off 'cause all of a sudden, jeans didn't fit as well and my thighs got bigger too. ... That made me a little self-conscious." In these moments of insecurity, Becky demonstrated resilience; whenever she felt insecure she would remind herself to focus on *all* of herself, not just how parts of her body looked or felt. She said that her mother would reassure her when she felt insecure that she was, in fact, beautiful.

Unlike most people's experience of university, which is one of a mostly sedentary life of sitting, studying, partying, and watching movies with friends, Becky joined the university's rowing team. Through this she became acquainted with her own strength and power, both mentally and physically. This is when I started to see the same theme that showed up in her mother's story show up in her own. Through rowing, she learned to treat her body like a fine-tuned, very productive, and valuable, machine. In order to perform best in competition, this meant eating healthy

58

whole foods, getting rest, and learning to find balance between sports and academic demands. Hearing about how much emphasis was put on weight for the women on her rowing team was a dynamic she was able to identify, and made me uncomfortable. It sounded as if Becky had weighed more, or had a different body type, that the focus on food and weight that came with being in a weight class type sport might have been a negative experience for her. This was the case for some of her teammates, who had to restrict food intake. Becky, however, was able to eat mostly what she wanted, and says that she generally got to enjoy her body, instead of focusing on losing or maintaining weight. I can't help but wonder how someone else might have reacted to this. I am so glad that this didn't change Becky's feelings about her body, but it reinforces that when our bodies appear to conform to what is expected of us, that we don't get the same treatment as people who don't "conform." Indirectly, this might have reinforced to her that if her weight was ever to change, so would the expectations of her.

Becky recently had a baby, and said that this has been another uncomfortable transition for her. But, like going through puberty, she says repeatedly of the weight gain and stretch marks, "It's not the focus." When I asked her to finish the sentence "my body is," she said very appropriately, "My body is healthy." And she answered the related question "women's bodies are" by mentioning, like her mother, the usefulness and functionality of women's bodies. The similarities between Becky and her mother were surprising to me, knowing that Becky had pushed against the closeness her mother wanted with her. I was curious about the relational distance that emerged when they moved back to North America, the distance that made Barbara so sad. About this, Becky said that her mother was looking for ways to be close and involved in her life, and at times this felt too close. She wanted to be her own person, and was learning—as is appropriate during teenage years—how to have boundaries. She found ways to protect her privacy and emerging identity from her mom, choosing not to tell her mother everything about her life.

She laughed when she told me about this, saying about her parents "they don't need to know everything. ... They were very, very hands-on parents, they wanted to know everything, and I don't think they needed too ... but either way, it's not like I have a lot to hide." I get the impression from Becky that she was a really good kid, just wanted to learn how to be herself.

In spite of this, she describes always feeling safe and cared for by her mother, knowing that at any time she could ask her anything. This struck me—she told me that feeling safe with her mother allowed her to focus on other things in life instead of worrying about feeling loved or not. She knew she was loved, through and through. This was meaningful to Becky, and she remembers that her mother's kind words to her helped remind her of her own beauty, allowing her to feel more confident and secure in herself, and in the world. Of her relationship with her mom, she says she "made me feel like really secure all the time, and definitely provided everything. ... If I ever needed anything it would be there, and that's true to this day. I really could ask [her] for anything and [she] would try to give it to me, not that I would take advantage of that, it just provides safety. I guess I could focus on other things and not worry about stuff like that. ... Instead of feeling worried about my family I could focus on school or sports or something like that." She speaks about her mother as a source of help, a refuge of sorts. Becky remembers her mother teaching her from a very early age about values, health, and the importance of family. And in her narrative, these are things that were obviously demonstrated, not just talked about.

One of Becky's strengths is her inattention to her image. She says of having a new baby, "Thank goodness I've got a mom who can dress, 'cause I'm not going to have a clue about how to dress this kid up." Although her inattention was and is probably helpful for her in some ways, protecting her from the depth of struggle with image most other women encounter, I wished for her that she would notice herself and her appearance, and take delight in it. I suppose if there is a hierarchy, thinking about your body like a well-oiled machine is better than hating it, but it's still not quite fully being *in* your body, and taking joy in how it looks and feels. She does, however, want to pass on to her children, regardless of gender, the skills she learned growing up. She wants them to be self-sufficient, able to cook their own healthy meals, and wants to teach them about how to care for their bodies well, like her mother did for her.

Some of the similarities between Becky and her mother were striking—it puzzled me that two different women, conducting two separate interviews without knowing what the other said, could answer the questions so similarly. They both spoke the same way about sweets, considering them to be a moralistic indulgence that needed to be rationed, and the focus on the functionality of the machine/body. Both women are strong, and come across in a "matter-of-fact" way to me. Becky does, however, have more of a voice of resistance than her mother. She has found ways in all the areas of her life to push back against things she didn't want, or like. This was never something done with a loud and aggressive energy, but she found her own private ways to take care of herself, and resist what didn't "fit" for her, whether this was with her mother, with culture and media, or in the demands of motherhood. It also made me think of this as being a telltale sign of the safety she felt with her mother. She was free to create space for herself because she was never worried that this would put her relationship with her mother in jeopardy. She could trust the safety of her mother's love.

Becky's statement was more profound, and psychologically significant, than she knew: knowing that she was loved made her free to experience herself, her world, instead of becoming preoccupied with fighting to earn love from her mother. When she said this, I felt like it perfectly captured what I was trying to learn about how all of attachment relationships between mother and daughter relate to body image. Becky knew that she was loved, and was accepted as she was, and that her mother (and father) would never leave her or abandon her. In fact, her ability to "push back" the boundaries she kept from her mother was not a sign that she didn't love her mother, but a sign of her own health, and how well her parents were loving her.

This reminds me of a principle of childhood thriving that I heard Dr. Gordon Neufeld speak about at a lecture in Vancouver in the winter of 2015. He spoke about the idea of the expression of affection exceeding the need: how much love is expressed needs to always be more than is required to survive. So, imagine that this entire time children's singer Charlotte Diamond was right, and when a child is growing up, that she actually needs four hugs a day to develop normally. According to Neufeld's principle, that the expression must always exceed the demand, you need to be giving her five, or six, or ten hugs a day. When this happens, not only is she getting what she needs, but she's learning that she's never going to have to "want" for the affection that's so vital for her life. She can become secure in her parents' love for her. Instead of trying to fight for that affection, she can use her childhood energy to discover the world, and herself. As in the times when Becky was trying to create more independence from her mother, Becky never had to want for love or affection from her mother. Becky had the ability to choose to move towards independence because she knew that she was loved—she wasn't scrambling to feel loved or cared for in her family. Another analogy of this comes if we imagine the relationship between children and food. Unlike adults, young children find it easier to stop eating if they are full, demonstrating their ability to listen to their body's cues. If there isn't enough food, and the young child is regularly starving, he or she will learn that if food does show up she needs to ignore the messages of fullness, because the time when food is coming again is uncertain. But, if the young child knows that whenever she's hungry she will be able to eat, then she can learn to listen to the cues from her body that tell her "you're full" or "you're hungry." When there is enough love, and more than enough love, we tend to learn as people that we can settle, and just be us in life. But when they're worried about if they are loved enough, and try and do things to earn that love, it takes away from what they actually need to do to develop in healthy ways as kids. This is related to the concept called the "hierarchy of needs" developed by psychologist Abraham Maslow. According to this theory, the more important the needs are for our survival, the more priority those needs have over other needs. We have some needs which are more primary, like shelter, food, and rest. When those needs are met, we can then focus on getting our next-level needs met: safety and security. I believe that the same is true in our relationships: trying to meet our relational needs for safety, belonging, and love can make it hard for us to do other things like explore the world, or ourselves, or cultivate creative expression. It seems like for a lot of people that is the case. We are so busy trying to survive, feel accepted, secure the affection in ways we never had it, that it is hard to thrive and be creative in all avenues of life.

LIVING FROM THE PLACE OF LOVE

I seem to always be coming back to this idea of "balance," when the mother-daughter relationship is working well, that it's not all black and white, that it's a mix of doing many things and feeling many things. For example, it's important that you want things for your daughter, and dream big for her, while balancing that with knowing that she needs to be her own person. There needs to also be a balance between stepping in and helping her learn how to see the world, and stepping back and just letting her form her own ideas about life. Above all else, she needs to know that you love her no matter what, and that love will never be taken away. I started this chapter by telling you the story of a woman I was working with in therapy who never got the chance to figure out who she really was. She had perfected the version of her that would garner her the most love and belonging from her family, but was struggling with what made life worth living when working hard to be someone that made her lovable and valuable to her family took away from her sense of self, and her ability to build a life that she felt was worth living. Although the early part of our work was focused on how to help her not end her life, she actually started to feel alive and enjoy being alive when we started to do deeper therapeutic work to help her feel and know she was loved and lovable in ways she never got when she needed it most. In this work, it was like she inserted assurance into her story right from the beginning that *no matter what* she was loved. This didn't happen overnight, and we didn't make all the wounds disappear. But we built a bigger and deeper well of love inside of her than she ever knew before, and that shut up the nagging voice of shame that drove her to feel like she had to be someone she was not. She was trying to be someone she was not, because she wanted to feel loved. And when she knew she was loved, she was finally free to be herself. The process of becoming herself wasn't as straightforward as she had hoped it would be—it isn't for any of us. As a recovering perfectionist, she had a really hard time with it.

I want for you to know what she eventually knew: you are loved. You are enough. You are no more valuable or less valuable if [fill in the blank here]. And when you know that about yourself, you're free to be who you are, without putting so much work into being who you think you're supposed to be just to secure that love. I believe that can translate to how you feel about your body. Your body is good, but your appearance was never meant to be the only way for you to feel lovable. If you know that you are loved, regardless of how you look, then you can start to live in the freedom that comes with not having to keep trying to earn belonging, value, or affection by looking a certain way. It might feel hard to read this, because I really don't actually know who you are, but I feel certain that you are more loved than you feel or know, even right now.

REFLECTION QUESTIONS

- What did your parents want for you growing up?
- What were the family and/or community expectations communicated to you?
- How might those have gotten in the way of you being uniquely you?

- If you could go back and give your younger self something she never got, and take out something that she didn't need to deal with, what would it be?
- What do you want for your (current or future) daughter, both small and big?
- What would it feel like to be praised for who you are, not just what you do?
- If you were certain you were loved, and you knew that would never change, in what areas of your life would that create freedom and healing? What would that change in your behavior, and where you put your energy?

▶ If you have a daughter...
- What are the family expectations that have been communicated to her?
- How might wanting that get in the way of what makes her uniquely her?
- At her age, what is appropriate for her to make choices about, and what do you need to make choices about on her behalf? When will that need to change?
- What is the best way to "get through to her" when you're communicating you love her?
- When was the last time you praised her just for being her, not for what she did or accomplished?
- What are some new or different ways you could show her you love her and support her?

FIVE

MEDIA: INTERPRETING AND RESPONDING TO IMAGES AND MESSAGES

"You do not win by struggling to the top of a caste system, you win by refusing to be trapped within one at all."

–NAOMI WOLF, THE BEAUTY MYTH

I had a book growing up which I loved and wore the corners of the pages off: a colorful cartoon-illustrated rendition of the classic Hans Christian Andersen folk tale *The Emperor's New Clothes*. Instead of people, the emperor and all the subjects in his kingdom were illustrated penguins. Innocent and playful, now that I think about it, it was probably a much easier way to get away with drawing an animal without clothes in a children's book than an adult male.

In Andersen's rendition of this tale, two salesmen approach an emperor and offer to create for him the most spectacular clothing. The catch, and probably what draws in the vain emperor, is that he is told that the cloth for the clothing is so special that it is only visible to those who are worthy to see it. The emperor agrees to this, perhaps feeling like this clothing would affirm his elitist position in the kingdom, and so the creation of the garments begins. The salesmen bring in a team to begin measuring, cutting, and sewing this fabric. But, no one can see anything, and in fact there is nothing there to be seen. But each person ordered to create the clothing, and every person who observes or supervises the construction of the clothing, is too afraid to admit that they cannot see anything at all. Admitting their inability to see cloth might mean that they are unworthy, or underserving. Terrified of being left out, of feeling lesser-than or being an outsider, everyone joins in, and thereby perpetuates the kingdom-wide illusion that clothes are in fact being made.

The clothing is finally completed, and the emperor is asked to try it on. His wait staff drapes him in his expertly crafted new outfit, and everyone holds his breath in anticipation of what will happen. Will he love it? Will it fit? Is it even there? But the emperor seems thrilled. At this point in the story, I wonder if he too saw nothing, but he had bought (with his finances, as well as emotion) into the lie that if he saw nothing, it was because he was undeserving of seeing it.

So, he responds enthusiastically, praising the work of the hands that created his new clothing. He pays the salespeople their extraordinary fee, and off they go. The parade for the emperor is set. In the coming days, he will walk throughout his land to show the people how special he is draped in his superior clothing. As the day of the parade arrives, all the people in the land have heard about this new cloth, and its magical properties. All of them, wanting to feel good enough, wonder what they will see when the emperor walks past them. The parade begins, and all the people in the town gather to see what the emperor is wearing. As he passes, the people cheer and shout, admiring how beautiful the clothing is. All of the people want to feel good enough; they do not want to admit they see nothing, because of what this means about them. At some point in the parade, a child looks at the emperor and shouts aloud over the admiration of the crowd, "But he's not wearing any clothes." By doing so, the child courageously says what everyone has known somewhere inside all along, but has been too afraid to say. In Andersen's tale, at this point the emperor cringes, finally having to admit that he's been duped. It is then that he knows that in order for him to feel superior, he believed a lie that ended up having him parade around the kingdom naked.

Whenever I think about this story, I like to think that if this whole thing really happened that I'd be like the child—the one to truth-tell, to say out loud what is *really* going on. And, I don't think I'm alone. I think we all would like to imagine that we're the brave one who sees things as they really are, who hasn't been duped, who hasn't been so concerned about fitting in. But if I am being honest, I'm probably more like the emperor or the townspeople—I think a lot of us are. We are worried so much about fitting in that we are unable to realize what we're trying to fit into is actually insanity. And, because the "fitting in" is a standard we've believed measures how good we are, we get caught up in playing along. Fitting in, being a part of something, is so important to us that we can get so easily trapped in a game of denying ourselves what we really know and believe for the sake of belonging.

Unfortunately, there are numerous parallels between this fictitious society and the culture we live in now. And this is true, most overwhelmingly so, for women and girls. The most obvious comparison I see is in how we are so desperate to try and feel like we belong that we will (either intentionally, or without awareness) shut off the part of ourselves that can think critically about what is being said to us, and how we often uncritically soak it up. We are so busy trying to make sure we "measure up" that we completely lose sight of how bizarre what we're trying to live up to is. Try this example: we see the bodies of women in magazines, and beat ourselves up because we don't look like that. When, in reality, the women in the magazine don't look like that either—the photos have been edited into oblivion. But, we keep buying the magazines, and keep shaming ourselves that we don't look like that. Where is the truth teller, the child, the person who will say out loud "he's not wearing any clothes" or in this case, "as women, we don't have to look like that," or "stop buying magazines that make you feel horrible about yourself." Until something is done and someone tells the truth, or we listen to that part of ourselves we have silenced all along, we will continue to be caught up in the façade of it all, clapping and applauding those who have achieved what we have learned to believe makes us matter, often secretly hating them for it, or hating ourselves for not being there.

It's not like there's no cost to this illusion either. I'd have to stretch the "emperor's new clothes" metaphor pretty far for this one, since the story doesn't give us much detail about what the townspeople are doing, or missing out on, while they're caught up in the illusion of the invisible clothes. But the real-life cost we have as women to perpetuate the illusion created by the media has serious, life-altering consequences. I admit that it can seem easy to blame media, if you are going to blame anyone or anything at all. And as I said before, blaming someone is a really tempting way to shift our responsibility. If I were going to say some of the things I just said, I wanted to make sure that that was an appropriate place to put blame, and that I had some proof for it. So I did some digging to find research that supports the idea that media is something that does have a massive influence on how we feel about ourselves, particularly making us feel worse about ourselves. Turns out, I didn't have to look far as the research about this is all over the place. In 2012, Fernandez and Pritchard[6] published an article, "Relationships between self-esteem, media influence and drive for thinness." Those are all fancy words to say that there is a real link between how we feel about ourselves as women, our desire to be more thin, and the media we consume. What these authors found out, by collecting information from 294 university and college students, was that the relationship between the influence media had on a person, and his or her desire to be thin, is really strong. This drive for thinness was true of both women and men. The next important piece of this study is that lower self-esteem is related to that drive to be thin. The way I understand it is to think of media as a cause of wanting to be thinner, which makes us feel badly about ourselves. I believe that it works the other way as well;

when we feel badly about ourselves, we are going to look for ways to feel better about ourselves. And, the media tells us that we can feel better about ourselves if we look thinner—that creates our fascination and fixation with losing weight, and for women to be "skinny." For example, when women are shown images (from websites or magazines) they are more likely to feel badly about themselves and their bodies, and say out loud in their own words that they would like to be more thin.[7] This was backed up by a number of other studies[8] which showed that not only is consuming more media making us feel worse about ourselves, but it can be directly linked to disordered eating, and extreme dieting behaviors. Here's the shocker to this all: the women in these studies who believe these things are educated, of many different ages and professions. And, in some studies, men were just as affected by thin-driven images as the women.[9] So if grown and educated women start believing these things, what chances do young girls have who take in images and ideas like a sponge? Is it easier for them to be "truth tellers" like the child in the folk tale, or do they have even more of a need than we do as adult women to learn how to fight the tide of images, videos, music, etc., working against their ability to be free, and loving of themselves and their bodies?

What I find most interesting about these studies, and our interaction with media in general, is that we keep doing things over and over again that make us feel worse about ourselves. What is it that has gotten shut off, or silenced, that as women we are so driven to measure up to the ideals set out before us, that we silence the part of us that realizes we're hungry, tired, competitive, lonely, and no matter how close to the ideal we get, never quite feel like we measure up? How do we get it back, or never lose it in the first place? Writing this, and rereading this, gets me worked up—I feel angry that these are questions I need to ask. I feel frustrated that we live in a world where we have to cut away at who we really are, how we think and feel, to try and belong. But I also sense my excitement and hope climbing up through my belly and out through my arms as I type. Maybe because we're asking these questions—as you're reading them and letting them climb in through your eyes and into your mind—maybe one by one and as a group we can we can start to heal. Maybe being angry about this is ok if the anger lets us push through walls and glass ceilings, learning to love ourselves and each other better, creating a different world one thought at a time, one "he's not wearing any clothes" or "she doesn't have to look that thin to be beautiful" at a time?

FROM FOCUSING ON LOOKS, TO REALLY BEING ALIVE

As a clinician and researcher these questions were of particular interest for me when I interviewed these women and their mothers. I wondered if they had to wrestle with the media, and how much it appeals to us all, or if they were never drawn to it in the first place, and in particular what their mothers said to the women about it all. The good news is that there were all sorts of different roles that media played in these women's lives growing up. No daughter, or mother, did it all perfectly. But, at the time of the study, the ability to see the media with eyes open and thinking caps on is a skill that showed up in each of the young women I interviewed. To varying degrees, they were all able to look at what is communicated to them through media, and speak the truth about it—in their own ways they were like the child in the crowd during the emperor's parade who said what was really going on. They all had different journeys to their ability to be critically reflective about media, but they had all arrived at that point. This is backed up by the research on this topic as well. Researchers[10] in one study found that when girls (fourteen-year-olds in this case) had a positive body image, they were able to be critical against the ideals of women's bodies portrayed in the media. They were able to describe these images as unnatural and unrealistic, and accurately evaluated the media as only showing one kind of woman. These young girls who loved themselves, and saw their bodies positively, were able to speak about beauty in more than just one, narrowly defined way—to them beauty was flexible and more than anything else, it was important for young girls to be themselves, instead of trying to look like everyone else, or what the magazines and shows told them they had to look like. Can you imagine if that's what you felt about yourself at fourteen? Or even now? Reading that study made me think about how much less time I would have spent on my hair, or asking for makeup for my birthday, if I felt like it was just ok to be myself. I've spent so much of my life just trying to get to the point of seeing my own beauty as it is, that it makes me sad to think about how many other things I could have done if I wasn't so preoccupied with looks for so many years. There is so much life to be lived for us as women, if we're not stuck inside staring at the mirror, or trying to diet. You have permission to imagine me climbing onto a soapbox for this last section. I really do think that we have so much to bring to this world as girls and women and that the never-ending chase of trying to look pretty enough keeps us from the fullness of our power, and the depth and heights we could reach in all aspects of our lives. If we could call out the lies for ourselves and for the girls and women around us that tell us we're not pretty enough, or being sexy means looking a very specific way, then maybe we can protect them from this incredibly unsatisfying and never-ending chase to be beautiful. If only we could believe for ourselves that we are already beautiful—even if our beauty is a different kind of beauty from the woman on the magazine cover, or the lady next to us at the salon—perhaps we wouldn't waste our lives away, and we could get on to really being alive.

TYPES OF MEDIA

Just to make sure we're all on the same page, the term "media" is really easy to throw around—so I want to define it. That way when you read and think about that term, you know exactly what I, and the other researchers, are talking about. According to a document put out by the American Psychological Association11 in 2010 called the "Report of the APA Task Force on the Sexualization of Girls," the media that we are speaking about here includes all of the following: television, music videos, music lyrics, films, cartoons, magazines, sports media, radio, the Internet, computer and video games, products (like clothing or cosmetics), and advertising. These all play a role in shaping who we are, especially since we are constantly seeing, consuming, and interacting with media all day long, even when we don't think about it. To emphasize just how much media we interact with every day, try and imagine your life without interacting with media at all: no social media, no advertising on bus stops, no TV, and no commercials on TV. Or, if in this imaginary scenario things weren't as extreme, imagine going on the Internet and no advertising pops up on the side of your computer screen, or no product placement exists in movies, or listening to commercial-free radio, or if you purchased a magazine and all that was in it was the articles you were hoping to read. The last time I was waiting at the dentist I picked up a magazine and for kicks just started to count how many full-page ads there were before I got to the article I wanted to read: I stopped counting after 50. Media is all around us, all the time.

SHERRY AND CARLEE

As I've said a number of times already, the women and their mothers in this study I've been telling you about all had different paths. So the good news is that no matter what you've done up until now it's not too late, and you don't need to start shaming yourself.

I want you to remember Sherry and Carlee, the mother-daughter duo I introduced earlier; Carlee is the hockey-playing daughter who always embraced the idea that she was supposed to have hips as a woman, and Sherry is her mother, who fought to protect her daughter against a struggle with anxiety that she had. There was a really interesting story that Sherry told me in her interview that particularly related to what she did to curb the influence that media had on her kids. Sherry and I were speaking about how she tried to raise her kids intentionally, and how different things are these days, particularly with media, than when she was growing up. She said enthusiastically, about the difference between her upbringing and Carlee's upbringing: "Social media, I mean 'hello,' we had *Good Housekeeping* and that's all that we had, and it was recipes." Emphasizing again, the difference, she said that growing up, there weren't large images of women on billboards advertising lingerie stores that are everywhere now. "I mean everywhere," she says. To further emphasize the point, she said that she and her husband try and stay away from watching television shows with sexualized images of women. He is a businessman, and she enjoys business as well, so they watch one of those popular shows where entrepreneurs pitch their ideas to big investors. Even on these shows where people are trying to get some investment money for their startup, she says that on "so many of the shows the girls are half- naked, so [my husband starts] fast-forwarding" through the parts where the women are dressed like sex objects, "and like seriously, we can't even watch those shows without these half-naked women, and they're beautiful, but it's like 'this is ridiculous.' "

Sherry isn't perfect in her ability to love herself just as she is, but she is able to do something very well—she is aware, and critical, of messages communicated through the media about women. She mentioned earlier in our interview that she didn't do any schooling after high school, so what she's doing well, she didn't learn in university and college. She may not have the fancy or academic names for it, but she can see that there is something wrong with what's going on. She, like that little kid who said "the emperor's not wearing any clothes," has been able to see media without getting caught up in it all, and say very appropriately, "Those women are not wearing any clothes." I don't know what it was like for Carlee or her siblings growing up with parents who made intentional choices about media. Maybe it didn't bother them. But there also might have been times when Carlee or her siblings were frustrated that they couldn't watch or read things that their friends could. That's normal when parents try and put boundaries on what their kids do. Belonging is a big part of being alive, so it isn't always easy when we lose something important for us, because of something else important for us.

DAD'S ROLE

There is something worth pointing out that Sherry mentioned in her interview. She said in an easy and almost unnoticeable way that her husband, Carlee's dad, does something very unique. Read what she says two paragraphs ago: on "so many of the shows the girls are half-naked, so he's fast-forwarding" through. ... Wait a second, her husband is fast-forwarding past the parts of the shows where the women are oversexually dressed? This man deserves a book of his own. There are some very important parts of this that need to be addressed before going forward. I think, most obviously, Carlee (as a daughter/young woman) is much more likely to get the message that women aren't just "objects" to be "ogled at" on TV by the men watching them, when she gets that message from both her mother *and* her father. The message here is unified between both her parents, which doubles the chance that she's going to pick up on it.

Try the alternative on: imagine that her mother and her father are sitting around watching a show and a semi-nude woman comes on the screen, and the mother says to the daughter, "As a woman, you are more than just your appearance, you are valuable for all that you are, and you don't need to be half-naked to learn that." But then the dad says, "I don't know what you're talking about. If she had something smart to say she'd be the one saying it," or just as well, ignores what the mother is saying and drops his jaw and drools as he stares at the woman in the bikini. At that point, the daughter may take in what the mother has said, but it's directly in competition with what her dad is doing. She's going to get her fair share of men who treat women like this in the world, but having a unified message from her mother and father about women's appearance, worth, value, and beauty will drive the point home much stronger.

In addition to the unified message, what I really like about what happens in this story is that Sherry and her husband are consuming media in a way that reflects their values. They are showing us that to interact in a healthy way with media, they don't need to get away from their TVs, radios, computers, and magazines. Rather, they have chosen that they want to consume media in a way that makes a statement about what is important to them. Their kids will notice this. Kids notice everything. In fact, two of the main pathways that parents communicate ideas and values to their children are through *direct communication* ("we don't want to watch shows where …") and *modeling* (actually changing the channel on TV when something they don't support comes on).[12] Direct communication and modeling are not just ways that messages about media are communicated, this is actually linked as well to how messages about food and bodies are communicated between parents and their kids. For example, imagine a scene where a mom says (direct communication) that eating food and being healthy is what matters, but sends the opposite message by what she does (modeling) when she sucks in her stomach in front of the mirror. This was something I discussed in the previous chapter about what happens when the messages we say, and the messages we act, are different.

PUTTING UP PROTECTIVE BOUNDARIES WITH MEDIA

As Sherry and I continued on in our conversation, we continued talking about the amount of nudity there is in the media, with women specifically, and how that may affect our ideas about women's bodies. Here is a snapshot of our conversation to give you a sense of the flow:

Sherry: We can't even watch [a business investing show] with these half-naked women, and they're beautiful, but it's like, this is ridiculous

Hillary: Yea, we use bodies, beauty, and sex to sell things, so if you're talking about business, well …

Sherry: But NO MEN, no men?! Like, I'll go to a movie and go, "Well, I've never seen frontal nudity on a man," but frontal nudity on a woman is like everywhere, it is everywhere. But not men.

Hillary: And especially like, oh, what's it called? [The popular lingerie store] and it's the large women, half-naked, blown-up photographs on the sidewalk.

Sherry: I used to get their flyer, and I wrote them a letter. I sent them an e-mail saying "stop sending me mail, I have a teenaged son and I'd really appreciate if you took my name off this list, this is not appropriate."

Hillary: Wow!

Sherry: Well, that was … I didn't want a son who … men and their issues with pornography is huge, and it's not cool. 'Cause, it gives us a poor self-perception because we [as women] think men just want to have "that."

Hillary: Exactly, and I think it's interesting you bring that up, because it's related to women's sense of self., We want to be beautiful, and not a kind of beauty that WE define, but a kind of beauty that we think other people want from us. If beauty was objective, then beauty around the world would be considered the same thing … long necks, or big earlobes, it's all culturally defined. And here, we've got a sex-saturated media, sex-saturated world …

So much happened in this short amount of dialogue between Sherry and me. We named together how women are treated as sexual objects in this world, and how it's all around us—even when we walk down the sidewalk, and what we watch on TV, but even the things that are literally put through her mail slot. I was so moved by what she told me about her desire to model for her children, especially her son, a healthy reaction to the sexualization of women in advertising. Not only does Sherry notice this about how women are portrayed, she took a step to change the level of influence that this kind of media (in this case, mass mail-outs from a large multinational lingerie company) has on her children. Her story made me wonder about all the other acts of resistance she has engaged in, and what her children took note of, and what might have just felt normal in their house.

What I learn from Sherry is that parents aren't able to control the world, and protect their kids from anything, or everything—this is especially true when children grow up, leave home, and experience the world on their own. But, we can make a statement to them, within our homes, about what we believe matters most, and in doing so, participate in helping to shape their ideas about what is healthy and unhealthy. What was also really unique about Sherry's action to have the flyers stop being sent to her home is that she tied what her son sees and interacts with (as a future man in the world) to the way women are made to feel about their bodies. When young men continually interact with media where women are thin, bronzed, plucked and waxed, and have perfect hair, it doesn't set men up to learn to love real women, as they are. When young women see men interacting with media like this, they begin to believe that they need to be like this too, because—as the argument goes—"men like 'that' after all, don't they?" So, instead of just trying to protect her daughters from these images, Sherry also took action to protect her son, as a way of trying to create a man with realistic and healthy ideals for what women's bodies should look like.

In response to that, I mentioned that beauty is something important all over the world, but if beauty were actually a very specific "real" thing, then beauty would be the same all over the world. But, we know that that's not true—women in other cultures are found to be beautiful because they have short hair, or have very large bodies, or have cultural and tribal tattoos all over their necks, faces, arms, and breasts. What this tells us is that we get *our* definition of beauty from resources, and narratives, and pictures, which are unique to our culture. And, if that's the case, then we can also choose to critique our culture's definition of beauty if it's unhealthy, or limiting.

This reminds me of an embarrassing story that perfectly illustrates this point. Several years ago, I went to the northern Philippines and volunteered for a number of months helping to deliver babies at a birth house. At the birth house, tribal women came to birth with free medical support they would otherwise be unable to access for a variety of reasons. I was planning to travel for several months on my own in Asia after my stay at the birth house, and was warned that this could be a dangerous and challenging experience as a foreign, young, Caucasian woman. So, in an effort to send a very clear message that I was not interested in being anyone's sexual bait, I grew out all the hair on my legs and in my armpits for the duration of my trip. I was hoping that if anyone were tempted to try and nab me, this alone would be enough to make them steer clear. As it turns out, leg and armpit hair doesn't mean the same thing in the northern Philippines as it does in North America. After some time in the birth house, a few young men had started hanging around, trying to get to know me. I couldn't quite figure this out as I hadn't exactly been trying to attract anyone's attention—and in fact had been trying to do the opposite. One of the younger midwives eventually told me that in that part of the world, most women can't grow body hair, so it was considered to be a sign of a very strong, and powerful, woman if you can grow it at all. Here I was, working hard to send a clear message that I wasn't trying to be seen as beautiful, but the language I was using to send that message was distinctly North American, not Filipino. Lesson learned. But, the point still stands: our definitions of beauty are influenced by different values and norms— ones which are directly perpetuated by media.[13] And with that comes the harsh reality that as long as we buy into the idea that that (what the media shows us) is the only way to be, or feel, beautiful, that almost all of us are constantly going to fall short. That is often usually followed by at least some amount of beating oneself up for having fallen short as well.

WE ARE ALLOWED TO BE BEAUTIFUL

I was giving a lecture to a group of students once about how politics inform our ideas of appearance, and what it means to be a woman. I was sharing several of the same messages I am in this book about the link between media and how we feel about ourselves as women, trying to remind that women are more than sexual objects, or how we look on our best and worst feeling days. A woman put up her hand, and while trying to conceal her annoyance asked if I was implying that women were not "allowed" to be beautiful. While it was clear at the time that she was being sassy, I think she acknowledged a tension that we all face as women: how can we appreciate and enjoy our appearance as an important part of us, without it being our identity? And, how can we enjoy beauty in ourselves and others without it meaning that we are objects?

Beauty—while most often used to describe an attractiveness in women—can be the word we give to anything we are drawn towards energetically, anything we think is ideal. Beauty isn't bad, and can be both something that we work towards or something that naturally occurs. It is a part of our world and is all around us and through and between us. But when we limit a person's value to how he or she looks, it dehumanizes the person, and misses all the other parts of beauty in who the person is. After further thought, the question this woman asked helped me distinguish between the beauty we naturally have as living, breathing human beings (including how we creatively find ways to express ourselves through our appearance), and the things we are told we should "do" to be a specific kind of beautiful that our culture dictates. If we *only* see "beauty" on the magazine covers, we are missing the beauty all around us. I believe that there is beauty inherent in all of us, and while our appearances can be beautiful, there are lots of other things about us that are beautiful. The problem is when we are focused on only looking for a certain kind of beauty, or when we reduce the value of a person (including ourselves) to appearance, not the beauty itself.

Thinking about this made me start paying attention to the ways I talk to and about other girls and women. It still makes my stomach turn in knots—I realized when I started listening to what I was saying that I would greet most little girls by saying how "pretty" they looked, or how beautiful their dress was. While I don't think it's wrong to acknowledge beauty, attractiveness, or appearance, I realized I wanted to acknowledge other things about little girls when I saw them. Even though I'm aware of all of these issues, my own difficulty changing what first comes out of my mouth when I see a little girl reminds me how early we start telling girls what our culture says matters most about us as women. I want to ask little girls when I meet them to tell me what kinds of books they are reading, and what their favorite subject is in school, and what they love about themselves, instead of just saying, "Wow, you look so pretty, twirl for me in that dress." If beauty isn't bad, but isn't something that defines the worth of a woman or girl, we need to do a better job of talking and thinking about beauty, especially with young ones.

MEDIA LITERACY

We can all learn from what Sherry does here: the unified message she and her husband send to their kids, but also her active stance of resistance with the flyers she received, to protect her kids from those images. But it's scary to think about how powerful and influential media is in shaping our views of ourselves, and what we could possibly do to resist that, both for children and for ourselves. There are a few things that you need to know first. There is a document put out by the American Psychological Association, which I mentioned earlier, called "Report of the APA Task Force on the Sexualization of Girls." This document makes some very important statements about media (I strongly recommend that you read it, so I've listed it in the references section).[14] It says that we can "not assume that girls are 'empty vessels' into which information from the media is poured but that they are actively engaged in choosing and interpreting the media in their lives, with increasing independence as they mature from girlhood to late adolescence (Rubin, 2002; Steele, 1999)." This statement is particularly powerful, because it reminds us that girls, that all of us, have minds of our own. If you have a daughter, it might be tempting to keep her away from things that are "harmful," or could be potentially harmful; the reality is that you are not always going to be around to do this. And, when you're not there to do this for your daughter, you want her to have the skills, on her own, to be able to interact with media in a way that's healthy for her. This is true about us as adults as well—we can't just run away from the things we don't want to see, because we'll end up walking down the street and seeing a huge image of it staring us back in the face. We have to have ways of thinking about the things that are damaging to us so that when we encounter them, we will know what to do and think. That is why seeing ourselves, and our daughters, as more than just an "empty vessel" is important; we are constantly interacting with media, and making choices which are reflected in, and a reflection of, how we feel about ourselves, and what we believe to be true about ourselves. So, the goal here is not to barricade her or yourself inside your home with no media whatsoever, but rather to help yourself, and her, learn to interact with media in a way which honors all women. This is called media literacy—it is the ability to critically analyze media in such a way that a person is able to "see through" the traps of what the media is doing, and be able to actively participate with media instead of passively consuming it.

Media literacy is a large part of having a healthy body image. There is evidence to support this as an effective tool for both preventing and repairing negative body image. In one study, college women who had media literacy skills were more aware of the unrealistic nature of thin women's size in media images, compared to those who didn't have the training.[15] In another study, high school girls with media literacy were less likely to internalize messages about the importance of being thin, and the unrealistic nature of thin images, compared to those without media literacy.[16] If you're a mom, media literacy doesn't necessarily have to be something you're perfect at before you teach your daughter how to do it; in fact, I imagine that it would be quite effective to learn about all these things with her. In my mind, I can imagine a mother sitting down with her daughter while watching a TV show and saying, "I've been thinking a lot about how I never look quite the same as the women on TV or in magazines, but I'm starting to realize that they all look the same, and all the women in the real work look pretty different. Have you ever noticed that? It's kind of strange and I'm wondering what you think."

"TRICKLE DOWN AND TRICKLE UP"

The "trickle down and trickle up" effect is a term I've borrowed from the APA guide that I've mentioned a few times now. It's meant to identify how women in media are portrayed to look a certain way—generally, something other than what they are. This process specifically refers to age, and works both in a downward motion (from older to younger), and upwards motion (from younger to older), blurring the lines between how girlhood and womanhood are represented visually.[17] In most Western media, women are made to look younger, or forever youthful, and by doing so they make real women aging in real ways invisible. An example of this is the women who are sexualized in such a way that they're dressed like schoolgirls, and made to look younger than they really are. In the other direction, girls are made to look older than they really are, posed, dressed, and captured as being older and more sexually mature than they are. There have been very publicized examples of this where preteen girls are posing for a semi-nude photo, or young girls are photographed in such a way that the prepubescent bodies appear to be presented like the bodies of women in their twenties. Next time you pick up a magazine, watch a commercial, or see an ad for a clothing company, take a guess at how old the girl or woman actually is, and compare that to how she is being portrayed.

APPEARANCE AND NONAPPEARANCE

In her numerous films and articles, Jean Kilbourne has famously identified that women of certain sizes, or races, are overrepresented in the media, while others seem to barely show up at all.[18] In order to become more media literate, we need to be able to think more critically about what we see, and also what we don't see. If you have a daughter, start thinking about how to teach her how to do this. You could help her learn to identify not just *what is* in advertising and other forms of media (for example, lots of very "sexy"' thin white women), but also help her learn *what is missing* (for example, older women, women of various body sizes and shapes, and races). While you're at it, you could even have these conversations with the boys and men in your life, turning yourself and those around you from passive media consumers to media criticizing powerhouses. You could even start playing a game where you try and point out media which accurately portray women. We also need to learn how to notice when images of women are edited and styled in order to present women in certain ways. For example, get familiar (and if you have a daughter, or female friends around, show them) before/after shots of edited photos that demonstrate that not even the model in the photo really looks like she is presented to the world on that magazine cover. Start paying attention to trends in advertising, such as images of women shown over and over again using cleaning products in the kitchen, but almost never changing the oil in a car, or chopping wood. When women are presented in the media in the same ways, over and over again, our visions of who we are, and who we can be, are limited to the narrowness that we see. I don't want to live in a world where being a woman means fitting into a narrow box of ideas. I want freedom, and opportunity. I want to live in a world where I can dream dreams. I want to exist in a world where I can live out who I want to be, and not choose what kind of sexualized and objectified version of a female body I want to be, or what kind of small, shrunk-down, apologetic version of a woman is least offensive to other people. I want real freedom.

OBJECTIFICATION

The term *objectification* is used a lot in women's studies and in psychology, and it describes how women are often treated or portrayed like objects. I remember feeling really sad, but also enlightened, when I learned early on in my studies about how we as women take objectification one step further, treating ourselves like objects: that's called self-objectification, when we turn our self (the whole person—mind, spirit, body, relational being) into just parts, or a thing. We do this all the time when we reduce our worth as women down to if our thighs are the size that we want them to be, or not. We also do this when we focus on making ourselves into a desirable object, to attract a certain person who is attracted to that kind of object. Objectification happens all the time in the media when women are minimized into things, or parts. For example, numerous advertisements will show only a part of a woman's body to sell a product: a pair of legs, or cleavage. Or advertisements will demonstrate a woman as a "thing" that a man can "get," not as a person who has thoughts, feelings, and ideas. As with the previous suggestion (what is shown, and what is not shown), it's important to realize this about media and help the other women in our lives, especially the young ones, do the same. Ads will focus on parts of a woman's body at the exclusion of others, and we need to remind ourselves when we see this that there is more to who we are as women than a part of our body. You are in this world for more reason than to be reduced to an object, or "arm candy." You have valuable things to say, and thoughts and feelings matter. Perhaps reading these words is the scariest thing you've ever thought of, because it might be hard to imagine that who you are could be anything other than how you look. It's possible that being so focused on being a desirable and attractive object distracted you from exploring and learning to enjoy the valuable things you think, feel, and have to contribute to the world. This might be your invitation to begin imagining a richer life, an existence which transcends how you look.

DESIRABILITY TO MEN

What if our beauty as women wasn't just "for" someone else, men in particular? For example, what if when we really know we are beautiful, it isn't because someone else tells us we are (or were) beautiful, or gives us attention. What if we could know we are beautiful even if no one else thinks so or ever tells us? What if celebrating our beauty isn't *for* other people, but because *we* enjoy it? The way that the media teaches us as women about beauty, and usually about the necessity of beauty/weight loss/fashion items, is that it will make us look more attractive. And, the goal of looking more attractive, as it is implied in the word itself, is about attracting someone else. The purpose of looking that way is for someone, and that someone is usually a male. This is a major theme in the messages communicated to girls and young women through the media—you will know you are "enough" when a man desires you. Through this we're teaching young girls and women that their source of value, worth, and identity comes from something, someone, outside of themselves, and how others perceive them. This is also reinforcing to women that one of the main purposes of being a woman is to get chosen. One term in the academic world for this is "costuming for seduction."[19] This implies that the way we should conduct ourselves as women (at least, if we're looking to the magazines and TV shows for what we "should" do) is to look and dress to get the attention of men, and be considered attractive to males.

What the media, and therefore the collective "us" in general, is missing out on here is reminding women that no matter what, they are beautiful, and good enough, just as they are. Period. Not more valuable if a man says so. Not more valuable if they lose five pounds. Not even if they are asked on lots of dates. Although there are many, a significant problem with this line of thinking is that as soon as they are chosen (if that does in fact happen), their entire sense of worth rests on the shoulders of another fallible human being. And that person, who is no God, but just another person, has been given all sorts of power they were never meant to have over another person. In addition to the dysfunction of making ourselves valuable based on the whims and preferences of another human being, it's also not healthy for the other person: it's too much responsibility for them to carry all of our worth.

PORNOGRAPHY AND BODY

It would be remiss to write about media and body image without discussing the effects of pornography. Pornographic images have been around for centuries, but it seems that more than ever before they have seeped into our mainstream presentation of the female body, accessible to anyone, anywhere. In addition to the unfortunate neurological, behavioral, relational, and physiological consequences[20] on boys' and men's sexuality from habituated pornography use, the popularization of pornography has contributed to a societal shift in the presentation and expectation of women's bodies. If we believe what we are told over and over again—what makes us valuable as women is being desired as a body by men—then what men have learned to want through pornography is what we as women learn to perform in order to continue being desired. According to pornography, what is desired is the same: one body type, one shape/size/color of the vagina, one style of body hair, all caricatures of the female body presented as objects for men's consumption. To get closer to the "ideal" or what we think men want from us, some of us buy magazines which tell us how to perform well in the bedroom, or give us tips on how to "give him oral sex that will blow his mind," while others of us get breast enhancements, vaginal plastic surgery, or dress in hypersexualized girl-like Halloween costumes. In her book *Pornland*, author Gail Dines writes that "media targeted to women creates a social reality that is so overwhelmingly consistent it is almost a closed system of messages. ... They normalize and publicize a coherent story about women, femininity, and sexuality. Because these messages are everywhere, they take on an aura of such familiarity that we believe them to be our very own personal and individual ways of thinking" (2010, p. 109). We think we are making choices about how to present ourselves, but we are acting out a story about being a woman influenced by pornography that we may not even be watching. The more that pornified images and messages become visible, the more normal they feel. What is driving this all is a deeply held belief that our worth as women comes from being desired by a man, or men. And to be desired, we presented ourselves in a certain "image." Dines states that "conforming to the image is seductive, as it not only offers women an identity that is in keeping with the majority. ... Looking hot does garner the kind of male attention that can sometimes feel empowering" (p. 112). When we are yearning to be valuable, or we don't know who we are and that we are loved as we are, it can feel good for a time to be desired by someone else, even if it's for an objectified, two-dimensional version of who we really are. The pull is seductive; it feels incredibly good, especially when we're feeling really special in a way that we never have before. So to claw our way back from getting sucked into this narrative, or to stop it in the first place, we need to have an equally strong counternarrative that reminds us of who we really are. In her book Dines writes about how women who resist sexual objectification proliferated through pornography and pornified images have an identity which stands in opposition to the mainstream, and they are not alone in this. Like so many of the young women whose stories are told in this book, being surrounded by other women who stand for this countercultural identity seems to be protective, and healing. Also like the women in this book, Dines notes in her work that the young women and girls who are able to resist the mainstream identity ("you're valuable when you are a sex object" story) have "someone in their life—be it a mother, an older woman mentor, or a coach—who prides some form of immunization to the cultural messages" (p. 113). She then goes on to say that what women and girls need to be able "to be able to continue resisting the dominant culture, is clearly a peer group of like-minded people as well as an ideology that reveals the fabricated, exploitative, and consumerist nature of contemporary femininity." Whether we watch pornography or not, or the person we are romantically involved with watches pornography or not, it has managed to infiltrate our ideas of what it means to be a female. It is abundantly clear through Dines's work and the stories in this book that in order to be healthy as women, to continue to refuse to be reduced to a sex object, to be used, abused, then thrown away by someone, we need each other. We need to no longer tolerate being invisible unless we are sexy to someone else. We need strong women in our lives, who speak the truth about who we are, and remind us that we are not just objects.

WHAT PARENTS CAN DO

At this point, it's ok if you're feeling a little discouraged. The world that we've saturated ourselves in is not exactly helping us as women, and it's shaping the way that girls and young women think about themselves. I always remind my clients in therapy that we don't really know how to be sad, or discouraged, well in our culture, but being sad in response to sad things is actually totally healthy. The APA guide I mentioned has some great ideas about how to contribute to changing the world, specifically for parents who want to help their daughters think critically about media. The first, *mediation*, is what you do when you get in between her and the messages she's receiving. Although this could be something you do literally (just imagine a heroic mother on a downtown street diving in front of a sexually objectified image in a storefront to protect her daughter), the in-between here is a figurative one. What this means is that you can actually change the way your daughter picks up a media message, by commenting on it in such a way that it makes her think about it differently. For example, imagine the two of you are driving in the car together and a bit comes on the radio where a woman is talking about trying to lose weight to impress a guy. Right there, in that moment, you could say to her, "Wow, that seems like a silly way to feel good about yourself. ... like, you can only really like yourself if someone else tells you you're good enough? Weird." Or, if that's not really your style, imagine saying to her, "What do you think about that? Have you or your friends ever tried to change the way to look to be liked by someone? How did that work out? What do you think the problems with living that way are"? By stepping between the message and how she takes it in, you're teaching her how to think differently about something that she might not have previously given a second thought to. The other idea is *co-viewing*. This often goes in hand with mediation, as it's much easier to mediate the messages when you're actually present with your daughter and viewing the same images. Co-viewing is just a fancy word for saying that you're present, physically and mentally, when your daughter is consuming media. This is why a lot of families choose to have TVs in places where families gather so that if something comes on TV that you don't want your daughter to take at face value, you can create a dialogue which helps her think more critically. It's pretty hard to mediate media messaging if you don't even know what she's consuming.

Like Sherry, there are also things you can do without her ever knowing—like canceling certain TV channels, or unsubscribing from magazines that you get in the mail. However, the reason we feel badly about our bodies isn't because our mom left one catalogue open on the kitchen table one time when we were seven. It's because the messages are everywhere, and we're constantly inundated with the idea that we have to look a certain way to be loved, or lovable. Even though doing little things around your home to protect your daughter is a good idea, it's important to start helping her learn to think critically about what she will encounter in the real world when you aren't there. This is easiest when you also have a strong and loving relationship with your daughter, and talk to her about all kinds of things; the more she knows she has someone on her side, who loves her no matter what, the better off she will be anyway. This bond that you create with her will remind her in those really difficult times that even though that person she had a crush on doesn't like her back, that she's not totally unlovable—your relationship with her is her proof. Helping her develop media literacy works kind of like a vaccine—when you get the injection of the "way of thinking," no matter what messages come at you, they won't infect you because you've been inoculated. Here's an example to prove it. In a study from 2011,[21] researchers examined three different groups: the first group watched music videos and ordinary television and commercials, the second group watched nature TV and commercials, and the third group watched everything that the first group watched (music videos, regular TV, and commercials) but with an extra commercial added in which showed the dramatic changes a model goes through to look as she "appears." This special commercial was intended to do what I had described earlier—mediate—and change the way that people thought about what they were watching. What the researchers found was that when the women in the study watched regular TV programs, commercials, and music videos, they reported feeling more dissatisfied with how they looked, compared to the other groups. Interestingly, the group that saw the special commercial describing how models are modified to appear differently felt much better about their appearance than the group I just mentioned, but slightly less satisfied with their looks than the group who watched the nature TV and commercials. What this research shows us is that even with a different kind of awareness-raising commercial, which is no match compared with the value of who you are as a mother, the women were able to preserve some of their sense of value and appreciation in their own beauty. Think about how much more powerful that would be if it was coming from someone they could interact with, who they could ask questions of, and have honest dialogue with.

THE TRUTH ABOUT MEDIA

My husband and I have an ongoing debate about music videos: he is an artist who also works in the film industry, and has always enjoyed how his favorite bands have carefully crafted a visual dimension to their music to tell a story. On the other hand, in my family home growing up I was never allowed to watch music videos. This was a choice that my parents had made to protect my brother and me from the oversexualization and degradation of women for entertainment. I haven't had cable TV since moving out of my parents' house after graduating from high school, so I was never really exposed to music videos at all, except when they've been on a TV at a restaurant, or an electronics store I'm walking by, or when I asked to watch them at a friend's house to take a peek at what I was missing. My husband's side of the story is that music videos aren't bad just because they're music videos. But, that in certain genres of music, the music videos portray women to be oversexualized, degraded, pieces of meat. Because of my limited exposure, I never knew that music videos could be any other way. One afternoon, he sat me down and showed me how one of our favorite bands had used puppets to tell a story reflecting the meaning in a song that we have loved for years. I got a taste for the first time in almost my entire life that a "something" I had feared would be horrible was delightful and lovely. It all had to do with what kind of that "something" I was interacting with. All of this is to say that media isn't bad just because it's media. We do, however, need to be able to pick and choose which kind of media we allow into our homes, while also educating ourselves about how to think critically about media so that no matter what we encounter, we can make up our own mind about things. This means when we see and hear things that cause us to question our beauty, our worth, our identity, and no one is there to protect us from it, we will be able to be like the child in the crowd in Andersen's folk tale and be able to know and speak the truth. We will be able to know for ourselves "the emperor isn't wearing any clothes," or most likely in her case "that woman is thin and mostly naked, but I don't need to look like that to know I'm beautiful just as I am."

REFLECTION QUESTIONS

- What kind of TV shows, magazines, and music are in your home and around you?
- What were the rules in your family growing up about what kind of media you could interact with?
- What kind of media did you see the significant adults in your life engage with?

- How often do you discuss critically with others the media you consume?
- What kind of media are you drawn to? What about others in your life? If you have a daughter, what about her?
- What might she be thinking about when she sees what's on TV? Have you asked her? Will you ask her?
- What do you want her to think about what's on TV? What do you think about what you see on TV?
- What might be some obvious ways to start questioning media? Is it easier to say something when you're alone, or with others who feel the same way? Is it easier to talk about really degrading media, or the more subtle messages?

SIX

STRENGTH: FEELING POWER
IN THE BODY

*"I know no woman—virgin, mother, lesbian, married, celibate—
whether she earns her keep as a housewife, a cocktail waitress, or a
scanner of brain waves—for whom her body is not a fundamental
problem: its clouded meanings, its fertility, its desire, its so-called
frigidity, its bloody speech, its silences, its changes and mutilations, its
rapes and ripenings. There is for the first time today a possibility of
converting our physicality into both knowledge and power."*

– ADRIENNE RICH, OF WOMAN BORN

When I was in elementary school, I wanted to play baseball like
my older brother did. At that time, baseball in my town wasn't
exclusively "boys only," but there was an unwritten rule that boys played
baseball, and girls played softball. But, my cool, smart, strong, older
brother didn't play softball, he played baseball, and so would I. Before time
for tryouts came, my dad and I would practice throwing and catching the
ball. I had my own (eight-year-old-sized) glove which he helped me oil
and break in, and we would watch my brother's baseball games together
on warm spring nights—talking about who did what on the team, and

who had good technique, and taking turns going to the concession stand for more licorice. Tryouts were held in a big school gym not far from my house, and to no one's surprise, I was the only girl who showed up. We had to demonstrate all the basics—and I remember every moment of it. It was my first "tryout" ever, and I was determined that I was not going to let my dad down. They had us sprint back and forth between cones, practice catching a ball, and in one exercise the coaches were on the other side of the gym rolling a ball across the floor, and we had to grab it and throw it back to them. When it came time for my turn to prove my skill, the coach rolled the ball towards me, but it was a little short—and I ran up to meet the ball and threw it back at him. I'll never forget when I was leaving the tryouts that day that my dad had his arm around me, and told me that I was the only one he saw that had run up to the ball when it rolled short, while some of the other kids had just stood there waiting for the ball to come to them, or for the coach to grab it to throw it again. My dad never said, you did well at that tryout "for a girl," or "because you were a girl." ... In my mind, and in my dad's mind, I was just like anyone else there—a kid who was trying out for the baseball team.

I was picked to be on a team I don't remember the name of now. Two other kids from my class at school were on my team, and so sometimes at school we would talk about games coming up, and what had happened at our practice the night before. But, a little while into the season, I started to learn from the boys on the team that I wasn't just another one of the kids who wanted to play baseball: I was a girl. And, to them that meant that I probably couldn't play baseball as well as them. There were several other boys on the team who were much better at playing baseball than me, and several who were much worse at it than me. But, when I didn't catch a fly ball, or when I struck out while batting, it was always because I was a girl, never for any other reason. I was performing just as well as lots of the other players. But, for some reason that didn't matter because I was a girl. I can't imagine that they learned to think that way on their own too, knowing the kinds of things that I heard them say behind my back—they were things that they had likely heard from older people, more sexist people, that they had picked up and said to me. One thing that they liked to point out in particular was that I had larger than normal hands for a girl of my age. This was something that when I was learning to play violin my teacher loved because it allowed me—later on—to play more technically advanced pieces of music with ease. But, when you're eight, and the only girl on a baseball team of prepubescent boys, I was definitely the easy target. I even earned myself a nickname for the size of my hands. For the most part I could take it all on the chin, but after one year of being up against the teasing and name-calling, I had learned that the boys didn't want me to be strong like them, or have grass stains on my uniform like they did. I learned that year that I could be tough and be like one of the boys, but it would cost me something. Even at eight, I knew I had better things to do with my time than be around people who didn't really want me there. I played lots of sports after that, but they were individual sports, or on a team of girls in high school.

Full disclosure, this is a memory that still stings with emotion when I talk or think about it, in both good ways and hard ways. But, I think that my story is like a story that most of us have encountered at some point as woman. As I sit here writing I can feel my chest fill with hope as I imagine a world one day where young girls could have a different story, or if they have the same story that they would be able to write a different ending to it. I was lucky enough to have parents who never told me I couldn't do something just because I was a girl (for an engagement present my dad bought me—*not* my husband, a tool kit with all the essentials in it). And because of that, I was lucky to be able to try something that most other girls wouldn't be able to.

But, I still had to learn that even if I'm ready to be strong, tough, and powerful as a female, that other people may not be ready for that, because it might threaten them. If for the boys on the team to know that they're more masculine and "manly" than a girl they need to be more strong, tough, and powerful than a girl, it might make them feel insecure if I'm just as strong, tough, and powerful as them. Before you rush too quickly into feeling bad for their insecurity, or maybe even questioning if I should be playing sports with the boys, why don't we blame instead the set of rules that limit boys and girls to certain things. I see those rigid rules as the real problem, in this case, not the rule-breakers. I know a lot of girls aren't ever given the opportunity that I was—to try out for the sports team I wanted to play on—because there are so many rules about what girls are supposed to do, or play, or be. And the backlash that so many girls face when they enter into typically "boy" or "manly" spaces—even their best is complimented in a backhanded kind of way. There is something painful about being told that you're "good at it, for a girl" that kind of takes away from the compliment altogether. It's a little like saying "that dress is nice, for an ugly dress"—where the compliment is really a putdown at the same time. Those statements feel more like "you will never be good enough, and no matter how strong your strong is, it's not that strong" than an actual compliment.

Because of these really specific rules, which influence practically everything we do from the moment we are born, we stop ourselves (or our daughters, or sisters, or friends) from doing things that as women we're not "supposed" to do. I do think that this genuinely comes from a good place; we're trying to protect ourselves (and our daughters, sisters, friends, etc.) from having the experience that I had—feeling like you don't belong, being made fun of, and getting squeezed out. But, by trying to protect ourselves and others in this way, we actually get put at risk for another kind of pain. This is the pain of not ever knowing the fullness of life, or the pain of having to make ourselves uncomfortable, so others aren't uncomfortable.

EMBODIED STRENGTH AND POWER
It is true for several arenas in life: we don't want to fail, so we don't try. Or we don't want someone we love to be made fun of, so we don't let them do something that is "different." Where this all ties together is that

experiencing physical strength, or power, in our bodies is surprisingly a really important element to loving ourselves and our bodies as they are. Unfortunately, this experience of embodied power is for so many girls something that makes them "different." Maybe no one is standing at the edge of the football field banning them from going to play, but socially and relationally, the message is enforced loud and clear: leave that kind of activity to the boys, it is not for pretty, desirable, and feminine girls. As you read that, I hope that it's all starting to tie in to what you've read so far. This point in particular connects back to what you just read about the media enforcing just how important it is for women to be attractive to men, and that anything which could jeopardize that could be trouble. This experience of physical strength and power can happen in so many ways— like playing sports, building something with your hands, or climbing trees—but a lot of times as women we're told that we don't do that kind of thing. Part of how we learned that is through the media. And because we were told that, we end up reinforcing that with our peers, and passing that message along to the generation that comes after us: the children around us and our own daughters. And these daughters, having heard it from most of those around them, either directly or indirectly, may start to hear it in their own heads, and feel it in their bones.

There are ways that these experiences in our bodies relate to how we feel about ourselves, especially our bodies.[22] And, it turns out that experiences of strength in our bodies, feeling the movement that we make in space, can influence the way we feel about our bodies. The opposite is also true—feeling constricted in our bodies, feeling like it's not ok to be strong and that we must not take up more space. This directional relationship can go the other way as well: what we *feel* about our bodies influences what we do in and with our bodies.

EMBODIMENT

All of this, statements about the self (which we usually think of as being our mind/thoughts/feelings/soul) and the body (the stuff people see on the outside that we dress and fill with food), can start to get confusing and deeply theoretical pretty fast. Especially since we're used to seeing them as separate, and here we are talking about them as actually being related; the body and the self are actually the same thing. While there are books being written about that specific topic alone, the reason it belongs in this chapter addressing strength is that we often forget that mind and body are actually both equally *us*. Take a second to wiggle your toes, or hold your breath for a moment after you inhale and before you exhale: each of those things you just did were all fully you—not just the neurons that fired in my nervous system to make those parts of me move. My thoughts are no more myself than the way that my legs crisscross when I'm sitting on the floor. Our mind and our body, together, are intricately interwoven, and together are all parts of who we are. This is why when we don't like our bodies, we feel badly about our whole selves. Or, when we feel really powerful in our bodies, we feel really powerful in ourselves. If our identity is just as much our bodies as it is our minds and thoughts, then we can use our bodies to help us experience power in a way that is just as important to the self as having thoughts and ideas or words that make us feel powerful. This idea is called *embodiment*: it's a concept that helps us understand and experience our bodies in a new and deeper way. Think of the difference between learning about a very specific French cooking technique, and actually doing it, experiencing it. Embodiment, as these ideas are formally called,[23] is the experience of being a self in and through the body, not just paying attention to what the body looks like. Practicing embodiment can help take our love for our bodies, ourselves, to the next level. Sitting at home watching TV, and thinking critically about what we see on TV, is a good start. But, that's the equivalent to reading about the French cooking technique—we also need to experience it. The doing in this case comes through physically being engaged in the world.

The mothers and daughters I interviewed spoke quite a bit, in different ways, about their experiences of being *in* their bodies in the world. To them, the most important part of their bodies wasn't how their body looked, but also how it felt to be alive in their body. Carlee and her mom, Sherry, who you met earlier, both spoke about how a focus on health and exercise was a big priority to them in their family. When Carlee started to tell me about the role health played in her family, she said: "My dad had cancer when he was twenty-eight and so, my family has always eaten very healthy. Because of that, I eat healthy, not because I would like to be thin, but because it makes me feel better, and it just makes for a better lifestyle, a better life. I exercise, I play hockey, but I do it because I love playing hockey, and it's good for you; it's just a way for me to get my aggression out." Carlee laughed as she said that last bit, about getting her aggression out, but then I asked her about how her experience with playing hockey shaped her view of her body, her experience in her body. She answered by saying this: "I don't know how [playing hockey] shaped how I view my body, I think it's just shaped how I view me, in the sense that sports empower me, and that I can be physical and I don't have to be like passive and submissive on the side like 'oh, oh, I won't go for the ball, you're a guy, you're going to come and get it.' I'm aggressive when it comes to sports, very competitive. So I view my body as I view myself as a strong person, like physically strong. Not the strongest out there, but it's not the size of the dog in the fight, it's the size of the fight in the dog, and that's what I've always thought."

What do you think and feel when you read what she said? Carlee's answer blew me away because she spoke exactly to what I was hoping to understand—how our self is a mix of body and mind, and how what we do with our body in a positive way can affect our identity. What is most powerful about her statement here is in how she hasn't separated her body from her "self." She says that playing hockey has shaped her "self" not just her "view of her body," and that in being powerful on the ice while playing hockey has allowed her to feel powerful in all parts of herself. In being powerful through sport, and having that experience of her body, she has felt more powerful as a human. It might be hard to catch in her answer, but she actually disagrees with my question, which asked about how playing sports has affected her body image. She takes it one level deeper and reminds me that image isn't everything to who we are as women—there is more to who she is than how she looks, or how she perceives her body to look. I think that in her answer she says back to me something that proves in another way that she isn't passive—she could disagree with me. I don't think her disagreement means that she is rude, or mean. To me it says that she knows who she is and isn't afraid to be that way. The immediate questions that start coming to mind when I read this are about how much we're missing out on as women because we're too afraid to do or say the wrong thing—disagree, play hockey, be strong and fierce. And, like I mentioned at the beginning of the chapter, we're afraid of letting others we care about do those things either. This happens a lot for girls. But, what we're really doing then is telling them that they're only ok if they behave certain ways, or do certain things. What we really need to be telling them is that it's ok to be them— and even more so—to be *more* of who they are; to dream bigger, to take up more space, to be stronger. That as women we don't need to be a less powerful/smart/strong/wise/joyful version of ourselves in order to be loved. It starts with what we invite ourselves to experience in and through our bodies.

GIRLS PLAY HOCKEY TOO

Carlee's parents allowed and encouraged her to be strong in her body: she and her brother played hockey together with her dad on the home-made ice rink behind their house. But, Carlee addresses how she also comes from a long line of seeing the women in her family be 'strong'. As women, we have a powerful ability to connect to other people, especially the women who have come before us, and after us[24]. By recognizing the strong women who have come before her, she has been given an example of what it could be like to be a woman in the world, in a way that she can see strength and power within herself. Here is how Carlee tells me about this part of her story: "I come from a family that on both sides there are

101

very strong women like my Oma ... and my great grandmother, and I learned recently that when she was younger she played hockey with the boys, like this was like yeah! right? And I heard that and I was like 'yea she did' right? I come from a family of very strong women and strong men ... also sensitive men, like my grandpa is so sensitive, he'll cry when praying for the meal ... to me a man can cry and a man can be strong and firm, it's the same"

It makes me smile when I read this part of Carlee's interview, because I can hear and feel the delight she has in knowing that her grandma was gutsy and defied the rules too. Her great-grandmother was a hockey-playing woman back in her day, which says a lot about her ability as a woman to defy the norms that were even more rigid in that generation. It makes sense that Carlee, and her mother Sherry, are powerful women—they were shown what that could look like by the women who came before them, instead of having to figure it out on their own. The image that comes to mind is of the old stone streets in Europe—the more they're walked on, the more the groves form in the stones and mark a path of where people have walked before you. The stones are less rough and harsh, but clearly define which way a person could go. I can imagine that if a young girl was trying to decide if she could play hockey or not, that if she knew her grandmother and great-grandmother had done so, even when it was more taboo, that it would give her the courage to do so.

It's also worth noting that she talks about the men in her family as being both strong and sensitive. It's clear from how she understands strength and sensitivity, that neither term is used only for one gender or the other. What a world it would be, both for women and men, if strength and sensitivity were not seen as mutually exclusive, rather appreciated together in the bouquet of the complexity of each human, adding intricacy to who we are.

Carlee's mother Sherry also played sports when she was young, and even when she had three little kids she made time for herself to be physically active. Interestingly, and like we mentioned before, Sherry's experience of her body isn't perfect. However, she speaks about being confident in herself from an early age, and that sports had a big role in that. About growing up she says; "I was active in sports... I wasn't self-conscious of anything." Even when she was in high school and she was a bigger size than her friends, she took pride in her appearance and chose to dress herself in a way that made her feel good about herself regardless of her size. "Most of my high school friends were thin, really thin" she says, "and I was never the tiny girl in the class, but I didn't ever have a problem with food, I was always active in sports, I think I learned early on how to dress myself and that made the difference for me." I can't help but wonder how hearing these messages from her mother, Sherry, influenced Carlee. Carlee got so much experience with being powerful, playing with the boys in sports, and connecting with her family through being active, that the dominant message she got about her body is one of movement, freedom, strength, and care. Even about food, Carlee says that she loves to eat, and that food is about giving her nourishment so that she can be more strong, playful, and active. I love the complexity to these two women.

STRENGTH FOR ANNE AND KELSEY

Not every daughter, mother, grandmother, and great grandmother play hockey, or sports together. Even though it looked a little bit different on the outside, the other mothers and daughters shared similar stories during their interviews. Kelsey and her mother, Anne, are another pair that we can learn from about this. You met Kelsey and Anne in the first chapter when I wrote about how mothers want to give their daughters a ladder out of their own struggles. You might remember Anne from her introduction; she grew up in a very abusive home where her father was an alcoholic. For this reason, in particular, Anne says she played a lot of sports just to get away from the house. I was curious. Knowing what is known from research about the challenges faced by adults who were abused as children,[25] I asked her point-blank what she thought made the difference in her life. She said almost without taking a breath that the reason she came out of such a difficult upbringing with so much security in who she was had to do with three things: sports, Girl Guides (Canadian version of Girl Scouts), and having a job. Being abused, by anyone, but especially by a parent, takes a very severe toll on a child's ability to develop normally, in all ways. And, it can have a profound effect on a person's ability to know and love themselves. But in Anne's experience, her activities outside of the home gave her power, identity, value, and freedom—all of the things kids are supposed to experience, but can't when things are abusive at home. What is admirable about Anne is that she had something within her— whatever it was—that drove her to get out of a bad situation. Some people call it surviving, or coping, but whatever we want to call it, she took care of herself, protected herself. She deliberately put herself into situations that reflected her worth, and what she wanted for herself in life—being part of Girl Guides and sports teams gave her the freedom and playfulness, as well as the experience of strength in herself (in her body and her mind) to get to know herself outside of the abuse. Interestingly, this also related to her experience of food. Because she and her siblings were playing so many sports, and her dad's alcoholism was so severe, sitting down together for a family meal was rare, and so she got used to eating hearty foods which were prepared in big batches and reheated easily—like chili and pastas. The message she got here was that food was for sustenance and was what allowed you to get through the day to your next sports game. Food was neither to be feared, not worshiped.

Her daughter Kelsey tells a really comparable story about her mother. When I asked her about her mother, Kelsey says, "My mom's life was very hard. Growing up, she participated in so much not to be ... to be out of the house, because her house was so abusive and such like a dark place. That's why she loved sports, but she was working, she was on every sports team, she was in Girl Guides. ... She tried to get out of the house as much as she could." The way Kelsey tells it, it sounds like Anne's experience of playing sports was out of desperation, instead of joy and freedom. Of her mother she says, "she did so [many] sports and activities, that she was able to see her body as strong ... that her body was useful but also something that could do good things for her." I find it amazing that out of her need to take care of herself, to protect herself from the abuse, Anne went to something that allowed her to feel her strength. In her coping, she found power.

KNOWING HOW TO REST

When I hear Kelsey talk about her mother's upbringing, she speaks in a way that reflects their closeness; she really knows who her mother is both as a person now and who she was as a girl. Kelsey has care and compassion for her mother in such a way that I imagine would make it easy for Anne to be raw with Kelsey—that as adult mother and adult daughter, they could begin to be real and raw with each other, like good friends—in a way that isn't appropriate when a mother is raising a child. Probably in a way that both stings and feels good for them both, Kelsey can see the gaps in her mother's story. Kelsey can see how being so busy playing sports, and being active, allowed her to survive but never gave her the experience of learning to rest in her body, and know what safety felt like. In a very gentle way, Kelsey says of her mother, "I feel like she didn't have time or energy, or there were so many other things like just taking care of herself, that she didn't have time to reflect on how she felt about her body, and I feel like in a way that carried forward." And that's when Kelsey identifies the paradox of her mother being able to see her body as strong because she was in so many sports. Here, she highlights an interesting nuance of experiencing our bodies as women—one that her mother never got to experience growing up. Sports and being active is important for us as girls and women to feel joy in the experience of our bodies. But, if we also don't know how to rest in our bodies—to enjoy a good stretch, the heaviness of laying down after a long day on our feet, the comfort of a shoulder rub when we've been tense—that the experience in our bodies is only one-sided. Sports are good, but we also need rest, and that gives us the full range of what our bodies are meant to feel.

I'm curious what you think about when you read that last paragraph—what parts of you applaud, what parts of you want to resist and push back? If—with a gentle and genuine interest—you ask yourself what you believe about rest, what do you learn? It's much easier for me to be still and rest than ever before, and I must say that I've been working very hard on it. Ironic as it is, I'm working hard to learn how to rest. It doesn't come naturally to me. But, the more I learn to rest and take a break from the ceaseless chatter in my brain and series of activities jam-packed into my day, the more I feel I come alive. Learning to rest means taking a break from all of the running I have done in my life, especially the running away from painful feelings. Miraculously, what has happened when I actually encountered those painful feelings and stopped the running is that I'm able to work through them. Then, in their wake, is peace. Peace in all parts of me.

MINDFULLY IN THE BODY

This can often be a problem for girls and women I see in therapy—they can "go, go, go" and accomplish a lot, but don't know how to actually be still and simply enjoy the feelings of being in their body as it is. I find that then there is a falseness to the joy they experience in their bodies, because they're not using the activity in their bodies to feel their own strength and drive, but rather to escape the experience of being alive, or still. Because, when we're really still, it can remind us of how much we actually dislike ourselves, and who we are in our bodies. If I were to paint a picture of what this is meant to look like, the active, engaged, powerful self and body, it would be done with mindfulness, or learning to live mindfully. Doing something mindfully means that instead of your mind being elsewhere, it's present with what you're doing at that moment; observing, aware, but never judgmental. So when you go for a hike, or go swimming together with your girlfriends or daughter, instead of thinking and talking the entire time about how many calories you've burned, practice enjoying the experience of moving through space and time, over and around objects. When you're lying in bed at the end of the day, thank yourself, and in particular the muscles and joints that make up who you are, for cooperating together so that you could be who you wanted to be today. Even the ache in your body after a long day can be something you respond to with gratitude, for the ache is a sign of who you are, what you did, where you went, and what it is like for you to be you. And you are good.

This mindful engagement with the world means that you're present in what you're doing, and not beating yourself up for what you're not doing. Kelsey seems to do this well—and she's found particular activities which beautifully engage both her body and her mind, helping her feel connected to all parts of herself and what's around her. Kelsey does this by gardening. She has found that gardening, growing her own food, is something that makes her feel in her body and her mind. She also feels united with the earth, and the circle of life and growth that we're all a part of. This has changed her way of seeing food as well, as she now sees food as life and connection, unlike what her mother believed about food growing up. She even spoke about how she would want to teach her daughter to garden, if she has a daughter one day. Kelsey reveals how important this has been for her: "It's exciting for me to grow my own food, and see that process. I think that was a healing process for me to be one with nature and watch things grow." To Kelsey this is a way to proactively secure a healthy relationship her future daughter could have with food, and create a sense of connectedness to self (her body, in this case), to each other, and to the bigger picture of the earth and life.

WHAT WAS UNSAID

The intergenerational piece was there for Kelsey as well, with her mother encouraging her to play sports and be active, like it was for Carlee. Kelsey felt like that was her mother's way of communicating indirectly that bodies are good, and can be strong and do work, and are made to be respected and enjoyed. She says that having her mother put her in sports "instilled the confidence that we can do well with our bodies." She doesn't, however, remember her mother ever saying out loud, "You are strong, our bodies are part of who we are, and are meant to be respected and enjoyed, and loved well." But there was a lot that was still unsaid about strength and power. She didn't mention in the interview seeing her mother play sports, or be very active, but she saw her mother's strength in other ways. The way Kelsey speaks about it makes me think of the same resilience that she described in her mother, about how her mother survived and got through such a difficult upbringing. I can't say for sure, but I wouldn't be surprised if being a part of sports teams, and being competitive—learning to enjoy working towards, or fighting for, something—helped her mother be such a strong person in terms of character. She says of her mother, "She's also a very strong woman, and will likely protect herself and stand her ground." This matches up with the quality I felt come through in Carlee's interview when she disagreed with me at points, and Sherry's interview, when she spoke with ferocity about sending back that lingerie catalogue. The way we might describe these women is that they're "strong women"—which, given what we're talking about in this chapter, includes both knowing their physical strength and their mental and emotional strength. Kelsey hopes to do what her mother did for her, but more, with the daughter she hopes to have one day. She, as already discussed, hopes to create a healthy relationship with food and the earth through gardening, but also wants to put her kids in sports. When she speaks about the important role sports could play she says that they "instill a sense that 'my body is not just to look good, but it can also perform and can be strong.' " But, she wouldn't want to stop there. She would want her daughter to know that the reason sports are played is because our bodies are amazing, and that how they look is only one component of us. Boundaries are also important. Talking about boundaries means teaching her future daughter about touch, eating healthy (what to put in the body, and what not), and how to take care of our physical body (including rest), so that the message she sends with activity is balanced by other kinds of care and love.

DEVELOPING EMBODIMENT

This fits extraordinarily well with the most current and valuable research about the importance of being active and physically engaged in our bodies—as it relates to how we experience ourselves. This is called the "Developmental Theory of Embodiment," and was created by Dr. Niva Piran, who has given her life to researching the prevention of eating disorders, body image, and how women can come to love to be fully engaged in who they are in their bodies. This, as I mentioned earlier, helps us get even further in loving our bodies, and preventing eating disorders. As women we don't just have hate or love our body as it *looks*, but we can also enjoy being *in* it. In this theory, Piran lays out the importance of three concepts that influence a girl's or woman's ability to be embodied. The first two I'm addressing at other points in this book—mental freedom and social power—but the third is the experience of physical power. This, just like our thoughts and social and relational context, is just as important for us to have a healthy relationship with our bodies as our thoughts. This dimension of our experience, our literal physical movement and how we take up space in the world, can be something that shames or constricts us, or something that makes us feel free or powerful. As I mentioned at the beginning of this chapter, we're often shamed or constricted because of what we're told by our culture, or other women around us, about what good women do or don't do with their bodies. For example, if a woman is told all her life that sitting still is a good thing, then she will never experience freedom in her body, and as a result, in herself. But, if she's encouraged to play sports, dance, and roll down grassy hills, she will come to experience freedom and power in her body, and as a result, in herself.

Piran gives us a few rules about what it looks like when we're doing this well. As I started out by saying, Kelsey is a real-life example of this freedom and power. Hopefully, this will give you a better idea of what this can start to look like when you're trying to help yourself, or your daughter, bring this to life. Physical freedom includes feeling safe, and having a sense of respectful ownership of our bodies. This means that whenever we do something, we intentionally take care of ourselves, and cultivate safety with and in our bodies, as opposed to hurting ourselves or denying that our body is connecting to the "us" that lives in our head. (This directly contradicts the experience of so many women, and in particular those who struggle with eating disorders, where it feels like the body is just a machine to carry around the mind.) Physical freedom also includes having freedom and ability in movement; this means that we're not stuck sitting with our legs crossed, hands clasped all day every day, but we can move our bodies in ways that we decided to move our bodies, and that we feel competent in our ability to do so. Lastly, physical freedom includes being comfortable with our physical desires, appetites, and changes that come with age. This means we don't beat ourselves up for feeling hungry, or how our skin or movements change with age, but embrace them as part of the story of our self and body in the world.

Take this all in: freedom in movement, safety and respect, comfort with desire and changes. Think about what that might be like if that that sentence was actually a description of your life. What would your life be like if you knew and felt all of those things in your body? And what would that be like if you could give that to the women you love, or the generation that comes after you? That might all sound great, but to me it's pretty terrifying. As a woman in the world, and someone who has struggle with each of those in different ways and different times, imagining trying to help someone else feel those things, and *know* those things, feels like a treacherous uphill battle. I really do believe it's ok that doing this might seem hard at times, especially when we remind ourselves that a lot of things worth doing are hard, and hard doesn't necessarily mean bad. It means doing something that we're not used to, and challenging what we are told, and the way we have lived our lives up until this point. It's never too late to change, and change is easier to accomplish when it occurs one small step at a time.

RAISING AN EMBODIED DAUGHTER

Think about how this might actually look when you're raising your daughter (and if you don't have a daughter, imagine doing these things for yourself). Try the idea of safety, care, and respectful ownership of a body. You could begin by telling her that as with all things or people in our world, when something or someone has value, we treat it accordingly. An example of this is we take very good care of a musical instrument, and we do so because it is valuable. The same is true of our bodies. And, this is why we clean ourselves, and do so with gentleness, and nourish ourselves with good food, and *don't do* things to ourselves that hurt ourselves (our bodies), such as take certain drugs or cut our skin, and why we *can do* certain things like get massages, and, take vitamins, and put lotion on our skin when it's dry. You can communicate to your daughter, first and foremost, that her body is her, just as much as her thoughts and feelings are her. And, because all of these things together are her, she needs to do a good job of taking care of them in a way that communicates to herself and those around her that she is valued. I can remember my mother doing this with me when I was sitting in the bathtub as a little kid, teaching me to take a soft wash cloth and clean all the parts of me that needed to be cleaned. Not with a vigor that gave my skin a rash, but gently washing in a loving and tender way. I have had several clients in therapy that are so disconnected from their selves, from their bodies, that they don't notice how harshly they treat their bodies until we start doing work on that in therapy. I have a special memory of a client rushing into therapy with excitement one afternoon to share the news that she all of a sudden realized, "Learning to love myself is showing up in how I treat my body, and care for myself, I'm no longer scrubbing my face so hard that it hurts."

The next idea, of freedom and confidence in movement, can look a lot of different ways, particularly depending on the context and who your daughter is as a person. You might encourage her to dance while there is music on in your home, and dance with you, even if neither of you are dancing "well" or in a way that would get you noticed for your exquisite technique. What you tell her when you do this is that being free is important, and she can choose how she wants to move her body, even if no one else understands. You could go skipping down the street with her, or chase each other around the park, or play hide and seek, even though you might trip, or look silly. You can remind her that she can climb trees, play sports, and that as long as she's not hurting herself or others, that she can be free to move in whatever way she pleases. If she is insecure about how to do this, put her in a dance, rock climbing, or gymnastics class. Or, better yet, do it with her, or teach her what you know. This will help with the competence piece so she feels she has enough skill to enjoy what she's doing—if we are doing something at least with mediocrity, we'll probably enjoy it more than if we're just struggling to learn. It's even possible that giving her tasks around the house which fit her ability and age could help her feel competent and free in her body. I remember a time when my chore one summer was to wash all the windows of the house, inside and out, first and second floors. I was terrified to get on the ladder but I had my dad hold it down below, and getting up so high and reaching to clean the windows on the second story made me feel so accomplished that I was beaming for days—taking everyone I could around to show them which windows I had cleaned. (Clearly, this had an impact on me; I'm still thinking about it.)

NOTICING, WELCOMING, AND TALKING ABOUT OUR BODIES

Lastly, embodiment means learning to be comfortable with desires, appetites, and age-related changes. This might be the most difficult part of embodiment to grasp, because it challenges directly what our culture says about who we are allowed to be as women. To be embodied means learning to welcome our body's cues, and invite others to do the same, noticing our hunger, thirst, exhaustion, and desire for movement. Being hungry isn't something to ignore, rather something to listen to, to honor, instead of hating it because it means we need to eat more. If you have a daughter, imagine that sometime in the future when she is hungry you engage her in a meaningful conversation about how special it is that our bodies tell us exactly what they need, and that when we listen to those cues, that we actually have a better, more full and healthy life. This can also be something you teach her, or remind yourself about, related to sexual desire and changes. If what you just read made you uncomfortable, I can imagine that talking about it with another person, especially a daughter, might not be the most enjoyable thing for you to do. As women, we do not need added shame or silencing for being sexual; there is already enough of that in the world. If I were to gamble, I might say that the discomfort you felt while reading about this, and thinking about addressing it one day, is an indication that you could have benefited from someone lovingly sharing with you about this. Just imagine how pivotal it could have been if an older, wiser woman who loved you told you what it was like to have your sexual needs met. Just imagine if someone, another woman, explained in a non-shaming way how our sexuality is connected to all the other parts of us, and taught you how to discern what was healthy for you and what was not. Just imagine how that might have changed your narratives around sexuality, and your own sexuality.

Learning these lessons is important, formative, and potentially even protective. In romantic relationships, if we can listen to ourselves, and know how to keep ourselves safe and respected, we are better able to say no to others when their actions are hurtful or disrespectful. We are also better able to advocate for our needs, not just doing in a relationship what feels good for the other person, but also knowing that our desires and needs are fulfilled Although these conversations might have felt uncomfortable on the receiving end if you received them (or maybe you were lucky enough to grow up in a house where it wasn't awkward), these conversations help us as women, and most of the time as adults we wished they happened more for us as girls and young women. If you have a daughter, think of how you can give her a ladder out of shame and silence around her body and sexuality, by having a difficult but important dialogue. And don't forget to discuss and facilitate the comfort with age-related changes.

These hard, but meaningful conversations are essential at so many different points of transition as girls and women: puberty, sexuality, pregnancy, child rearing, menopause and later, aging. Even if we don't have a mom we can talk to about it, or if we don't have a daughter to pass on our wisdom to, we need each other as women when things are changing. Even if things are hard, or scary, having people to talk to who are going through the same changes, or have been through them before, reminds us that we're human, and not alone. Not surprisingly, what we talk about when we have these hard conversations matters too, especially when we're sharing experiences with those who will come after us. What we tell girls and younger women about these big transitions can create fear and shame. We all need to know that what we're experiencing is hard, but normal, because whenever we're going through something for the first time, we don't know what's normal, because it's all different and more uncomfortable than what we knew before.

If you have a younger woman in your life, a daughter perhaps, it might be hard to imagine having conversations about all these things, especially if no one ever had them with you. And when the experiences you have had with a changing body haven't exactly been positive, then I could imagine it might feel phony to tell her anything other than your war stories. To some degree, that's helpful. It will remind her that the first time during her period that she bleeds through her underwear (and pants) she is not the first female in history that that has happened to. If you don't have a daughter, take a moment to remember the significant moments and periods of time when lots of change was happening in your body. Try and remember what it was like, and if you could go back and talk to your younger self at those moments, what you would want her to know.

Whether it's a daughter, a future daughter, a niece, or your younger self, imagine this: Celebrate the transition to puberty by reminding her that this is an important step in her journey towards womanhood. You can remind her that when she ages, the lines and wrinkles on her face tell the stories of what she's felt, how she's laughed, and what's she's been through. You, like the women I've been telling you about, can tell her that she has the most miraculous ability to bear life, and with that comes some things like bigger hips, more fat, and the gift of caring and nurturing others. Those are not things that need to define her, but she can enjoy them and look forward to changes in her body, as she ages, because they connect her to the beautiful and powerful story of womanhood. Even cellulite, something most women fear and try and rid their bodies of, is just a normal mark of how the female body stores fat, and is nothing that will ever make her less lovable or beautiful.

Perhaps it might seem more far off than possible at this point, but I believe that when we tell the next generation of women (and ourselves at the same time) that all the changes they are going to go through are not awful but actually normal, important and even beautiful, we might be able to eradicate from the next generation of girls and women the shame that we have learned to feel about ourselves in our bodies.

PRACTICING EMBODIMENT

A renown psychologist named Dr. Peter Levine specializes in using the body to help us heal psychologically. Most of us, and especially individuals who have suffered trauma, experience ourselves outsides our bodies, or a divide between our minds and our bodies. In one of his books, *Waking the Tiger*,[26] he has an exercise that might be useful for you to try to help you experience embodiment. Take time to have a shower where you do not have to rush off to anything, with the showerhead on pulsing if possible. Make sure the temperature is cool or slightly warm. Move your body under the pulsing water and stay there for a moment. See if while you are there you can draw all of your conscious awareness into that part of your body. As you move body parts under the pulsing water, let your focus shift. Try doing this with every part of your body, and when you are doing it say to yourself "this is my head," "I am here, in this moment," or 'welcome back." In doing this, Levine reminds us about how this reconnects our sense of self, our mind, back to our bodies. It is through moments like these in the shower that we can start to build a more embodied existence, reminding ourselves—or learning for the first time—how good it is to be us.

IF OUR BODIES WERE NOT THE SOURCE OF SHAME

A few years ago my mom and I were at a big theatre downtown to see a musical we had wanted to see together for almost a decade. At the intermission we were waiting in the impossibly long line for the bathroom and I told her about a book I was reading called *When Women Were Birds*, by Terry Tempest Williams. In this particular vignette she tells the story of her first period. It will always stick with me. I do still think of it often, as both a painful pushing on a bruise of something I wish I had, as well as the beacon for which I hope we can strive when helping to shape the relationships that the next generation of women have with their bodies. The excerpt, in its entirety, is as follows:

> *"When my period came for the first time, I called my mother from school. I was in the eighth grade.*
>
> *"'It's here,' I said.*
>
> *"'I'll be right there,' she replied.*
>
> *"Once home, she made me a bath of rose petals."*

Even now as I read it, I feel my eyes begin to tear. Her story is so different than my experience of my first period, for which I felt so much shame and confusion that I literally never spoke of it, but told my mom in a note I left under her pillow. We had no discussion, no celebration, no shared story of what this means, why it is scary and good all at once, and something to be experienced with honor. My experience is so different than what I hope to give my daughter one day as a rite of passage into womanhood. It is so different than what I hope for myself for all of the times I tell the people in my life about something new and scary and confusing. And it is so different than how I hope to respond when the women in my life take the risk to share their raw and vulnerable self with me. As my mother and I stood in the lineup for the bathroom at the big fancy theatre, our eyes became blurry with tears. She put her hand around my shoulder and I knew she was with me, and understood. We have had many moments of silence in our relationship, where all of my shame and fear bottled up in my throat and got in the way of me naming the things that were happening for me. I'm sure it was the same for her. Shame, and the fear of what will happen when we risk, does that to us. But it is not lost on me that I could finally tell her. I know some women will never have the chance, or it will never be safe for them to tell their mothers how they needed them, and how much it hurt that they weren't there. Although likely strange-looking to the other women casually waiting in the lineup, the silence and the divide continued to heal that day.

What Williams' mother told her was that her body was good, and is good, and is actually something not to be feared, shamed, or silenced, but something to be celebrated, honored, and enjoyed. Even with menstruation, something that is often dreaded, we can rejoice in this being something our bodies do as part of the poetry written into our biological, and relational, narratives as women.

As with a first period, joining a sports team, and how we sit at the dinner table, we have the ability to cultivate in ourselves, and in our daughters, the experience of power, strength, and freedom. We are our bodies. Our skin is just as much "us" as our heartbreak. We are just as much our liver and pancreas as the "self" that sings along to the music on the radio, or gives gifts to loved ones. We are just as much the softness of our eyelashes, as the ways we laugh or tell jokes, or not. The freedom and power available in and through our bodies is for all of us, no matter our age, what kind of body-baggage our mother has, what size we are, how we have felt about our body in the past, or what others think or say. Freedom, power, and strength is ours for the taking.

REFLECTION QUESTIONS

- When was the last time you felt the power of your body, and enjoyed being in your body?
- When was the first time you felt that way?
- What might you be telling your daughter about her body, without meaning to, about what it means to be a girl, or to be strong?
- What do you think when your body tells you something? How do you normally respond to fatigue, hunger, thirst, sexual desire, shivering, or sweating?
- If you have a daughter, would you like to communicate to her about these things?
- What do you wish was said to you, when you were younger, about your body?
- What could you do with your daughter, as an activity, to engage in play and freedom and strength of the body, together?
- When do you feel most powerful in your body? What is that like for you? Do you remember how that has changed over the course of your life?
- Who are the strong women in your family? How are they strong? How are you like them?
- Who are the strong women around you in your life right now?

SEVEN

RELATIONAL SELVES: VOICE, MENTAL FREEDOM, AND SOCIAL POWER

"And the day came when the risk to remain tight in a bud was more painful than the risk it took to blossom."

-ANAÏS NIN

One of the numerous unwritten rules of femininity is that we are "never" allowed to tell another girl or woman, especially an equal—someone we respect and feel close to—that she is, or looks, fat. Think about it: if a girlfriend of yours asked you if she looks fat in her jeans, your heart would not even beat once before you coolly responded with a "no way" or "You? Not a chance." Never would you tell that friend, "I notice you have put on some extra weight recently and I'm concerned about your health," or "What has changed in your life that might be affecting how you treat yourself?" This idea—telling someone what they want to hear, not what's true—translates to so many, perhaps all, other spheres of our lives as women. If a friend is dumped, you're likely to say, "I never liked 'so and so,' " or, "That person was no good for you." Rarely, if ever, would you ask that friend to consider what she might have done to be responsible, at least in part, for what happened between her and that former partner.

Boil it all down, and for the most part, there's a code by which we live our lives as women: don't say what you actually think or feel, say what the other person wants you to say and wants to hear. Don't create conflict, don't make anyone uncomfortable, and don't ever say no. Be yourself, but only if being you includes being "good" or nice and nonconfrontational. This isn't the way it always was for us. And, there's proof that as we grow up from girls to women we all get to a critical point when we start to learn it's not ok to be us anymore, and that we need to start being what other people expect of us.

Recently, a friend told me that when her daughter was younger, she looked at a woman in front of them in line at the grocery store and pointed to her face and said out loud, "Mom, that lady has a moustache." That little girl was just saying what she knew to be true, and was also really proud of saying something out loud that she had just learned. Everyone in that grocery store probably thought it, but that little girl hadn't learned yet that some people don't like the truth being said out loud. All the memories amalgamate in my mind, but I can remember in elementary school my friends and I saying out loud to each other what we thought. "You hurt my feelings, I'm upset with you," or "Why aren't you sharing with me, but you're sharing with her?" were normal things to be said and heard on the playground in those early years. As girls, most of us haven't "unlearned" yet how to say what we really feel.

RELATIONAL SELVES
In my second year of university, I was introduced by my psychology of gender professor to some groundbreaking psychological research, conducted by some very smart and gutsy women at the end of the 20th century.[27] These women (Carol Gilligan, Mary Field Belenky, Jean Baker Miller, and others) were redoing some of the classic psychological studies on moral development; how people determine what is right and

wrong. These female scholars had noticed that the major studies done on morality and development were done by researching boys and men—no girls or women in the studies at all. But the findings were extrapolated to women just the same. So, these gutsy researchers started to redo some of the studies, asking girls and women the same questions as in the earlier studies. And, they came across the same phenomenon I just mentioned that somewhere in the process of growing up, women were no longer telling the truth about what they thought and felt in the way that the girls in the studies did. Thinking about that still blows my mind; the thing that we all do as women (trying to being what others expect) wasn't always that way in our lives, and doesn't have to always be that way. It's something we learn. What the researchers concluded was that this shift, from knowing who you are and what you think and feel, to trying to be what is expected of you, takes place sometime around puberty. It happens around the same time that girls start to notice that their bodies are changing, and boys are noticing them (or not), and that how they feel about themselves might be shaped by how other people see them. This is a well-developed idea in psychology, and women's studies, which identifies that women are relational beings. What this means is that we see ourselves in the context of our relationships, not just as islands or lone rangers accomplishing individual tasks. We identify ourselves, and often consequently our worth, by the quality of our relationships we have with others. This includes how we are seen, or believe ourselves to be seen, through the eyes of others particularly those we're in relationships with or those we deem important.

This can be one of the most beautiful, and fruitful, dimensions of our lives as women; the experience of connectedness that comes from desiring relationships with others is something that will always make our life richer, and rarely lonely. It's something many men miss out on because of what our culture tells them about what it means to be a man: don't show emotion, don't be vulnerable, don't need others. In fact, it is through relationship that we can come to know more of ourselves. This makes me think about a time recently when I went to the house of one of my best friends, and while Alexandra made us dinner I talked and talked and talked. I shared with her some things that had happened that week which had left me feeling unsettled. She asked questions, and stayed engaged with me the whole time, walking me through how she saw what happened, in a way that helped me come to understand why I might have felt what I felt. In being empathetic with me ("I would feel frustrated if that happened to me too") it reminded me that I—and my feelings—were safe with her and what I was experiencing was a normal part of the human experience. She happens to be a very wise, and skilled, social worker, so it was probably as close to therapy as I could get without actually doing therapy. But in being honest and raw with her, I came to know myself and learn about myself more. There are hundreds of examples of this, and I know I'm lucky to have her, but our deep bond is a function of both of us showing up with each other, and being authentic. In moments of vulnerability, I have done my work to share with her my deepest fears and shame, and she has done her part: staying present with me emotionally, with arms wrapped around me while I cried. It is through relationship with her that I can come to know and love myself more, finding my voice, and learning to love it through the safety of my relationship with her. What is most special about letting ourselves be seen by people who are willing to have this kind of relationship with us is that we can have a repair of the self. When we risk to let ourselves be seen, the real us, and we have someone love us and care for us, we are reminded that we are loved and lovable just as we are—not as who others expect us to be.

This part of our relational selves is also what makes it so easy for us to care for others, and enjoy sitting around for hours just talking. Dr. Jean Baker Miller, a specialist in women's psychology, says "to feel more related to another person means to feel one's self enhanced, not threatened. It does not feel like a loss of part of one's self, instead it becomes a step towards more pleasure and effectiveness."[28] When we connect to others, we don't have to lose a part of ourselves; we can actually gain a part of our selves. Through meaningful connection, we become more fully ourselves.

We can celebrate this dimension of who we are as women. As you consider your own experience as a woman in the world, we also need to consider that this rationality which is so central to who we are can also be something which hurts the development of a healthy self. Being relational means that at times we can overemphasize the importance of relationships, to the point where we actually diminish our ability to be an individual. There is even research that identifies that the important role relationships play in our development as women can get in the way of a girl's ability to be healthy as a self.[29] As humans, it can often feel as if these things are in conflict with each other, balancing what it means to be a person who is also relational. And sometimes we get a glorious moment of feeling like we get to be connected to someone just as we are—to me that is when I feel most fully alive, and like I'm healing. The emphasis on relationships, especially among adolescent girls, can make a girl feel more self-conscious, wondering a lot of the time what other people think of her. This is directly related to how a preteen or teenage girl then thinks about herself inside her head. You might remember this from your adolescence, spending far too much time reading into what other people might be thinking about you, and becoming more vulnerable to the opinions of others.[30] The more fragile the relationships, or the girl's sense of self-worth, the more likely it was that she was going to push down what she really thought and felt, in order to be liked by others. Carol Gilligan, one of the main authors of the studies I have mentioned, identified this as "loss of voice": the way that we as girls and women learn to suppress our thoughts and feelings to prevent conflict. Loss of voice is also known as "silencing the self"– which does a better job of identifying that we are actively keeping something down, instead of just having misplaced it at some point during our daily chores, like losing our keys or glasses.[31] Although, after having silenced something for so long, over and over again, shutting down the things we want and feel, it's possible that it might seem like it really is gone, lost forever. What's both fascinating and terrifying about this is that this loss of voice has been linked to depression and the development of eating disorders.[32] It all comes full circle. That is why knowing ourselves and having a voice is important to loving our bodies, and paving the way for young women to do the same. Our voice, both literally and metaphorically, like our body, is an important part of who we are. Together our voice and our body are bridges through which other people can join us in connection, and they represent some of the important aspects of who we are, and what it means to be us in the world.

WHAT OTHERS EXPECT, AND WHO WE REALLY ARE

Here's a story to further illustrate the point: a client who I've been working with concerning her self-esteem told me about how she really only feels good enough about herself if her friends tell her they like what she's wearing. She has been depressed, and been a chronic dieter for most of her life. When she became a mom, she wasn't with her friends as much, so felt like her self-worth plummeted. Her favorite clothes didn't fit, and she didn't have people around all the time to tell her they liked how she looked. She came into therapy one afternoon feeling an immense amount of distress; she was planning on going out with her girlfriends and found herself obsessing over what she would wear even two weeks prior to when they were planning to get together. Her entire ability to be "ok" rested in the hands of the people around her. And, in what they thought about how she looked. She eventually went out to buy an outfit more expensive than she could afford, just to make sure that when they saw her, she knew they would tell her how great she looked.

The focus we put on our looks as women, and how that plays out in our relationships, all converge in that one woman's story. Interestingly enough, so does the part I've been mentioning about "what she thinks other people want her to say." When she came into my office, and told me about the upcoming event, how she had obsessed about her outfit, then bought new clothes, she told me how embarrassed she was to have to admit that to me, because she thought she knew what I would want her to say. I asked her what she thought I wanted her to say. She said, "I think you want me to say that I don't care what my friends thought and wore what I wanted to wear because I wanted to wear it." She smiled at me sheepishly, nervous of how I would react. I felt sad in that moment. I want her to *know* that she is enough, just as she is, and not simply trick herself into thinking that so she can be who I want her to be. I paused for a moment, knowing in a more obvious way now that I have to encourage her to be more fully her, not more fully me. I told her about how much I admired her bravery with me, telling me about her inner conflict about if to tell me the truth, or what she thought I wanted to hear. Although I wish for her, and for us all, the freedom from feeling like we're defined by our appearance, I also deeply admired the risk she took to tell me the truth about herself, and her choice in our session to show me the *real* her. I wanted her to know that we can only do real work when we allow ourselves to encounter our real self, and that in our therapy together that I would never shame her, or judge her, when she let me see the most vulnerable parts of her.

I remember in that moment how scared she must have been, caught in between what she felt she really wanted—to know she was good enough in the eyes of her friends—and to know from me that she was doing a good job. Just like the approval from her friends, she wanted approval from me. She did, however, have the courage to be honest with me about what was going on, and was able to see as we worked through it that I want her to get better at loving herself for her sake, and because she knows she is worth it, not just because I tell her that's what she has to do. In our work together we spoke often about what it's like if we don't balance being relational with knowing who we are as an individual; we can get pulled into an unhealthy balance of trying to do just one or the other. But, to be healthy as girls and women, we need both. We cannot forsake who we are, and who we are as both a unique individual and person who is wired for connection and relationship. We will always be most ourselves when they are both in balance.

This balance of both, being relational and knowing who we are as an individual, is hard in a world where we're reinforced for being who others want us to be. Often, when we are who they want us to be, we get reinforced that this is a wonderful thing, and we feel good, for a time. But, that wears off. So, we start to do more things for other people to make ourselves feel good again. After a while, an authentic self doesn't exist in those relationships anymore, and we are only loved and valued for being what another person wants us to be, not for being truly ourselves. For a long time, I had a very hard time saying "no"' to anyone who asked for anything, especially if what they asked for was something that I valued too, like helping, building someone up, or reminding them that they're not alone in this world. I've had to learn, in the course of having my own practice as a therapist, that even though it would really help a client, or coworker, to take their friend of a friend or relative on as a client, I can only help so many people before I actually stop enjoying what I do, or stop doing it well enough that I'm not actually helping people. I feel like it's wrong for me to preach balance and self-care all day long, and then never practice it myself: it's a work in progress. But the part of ourselves that wants to care for everyone else can become a dangerous trap. When I'm feeling down on myself, or like I am not a particularly valuable person, but I squeeze one more client in on a long day, and they thank me and tell me a hundred times how amazing I am, I start to feel better about myself. And so the beast of proving and fixing is fed. I can't tell which comes first, the loss of self, or the praise we get from others when we are giving in a way that benefits them, but they are certainly related. This has a cost. So, too, does denying those around us, and only thinking about ourselves. Either one or the other creates a life that neglects one part of who we are as a woman, and keeps us from being whole.

HELPING YOUR DAUGHTER HOLD ONTO HER VOICE

(If you don't have a daughter, try reading this next section and reflect on what your mother did, or didn't do, related to the development of your voice. You could also think of the young girl part still alive inside of you who needs you to mother her in the way your own mother never did.)

This all translates directly to how you, as a mother, play a valuable role in raising a daughter who loves herself, and her body, as is. At several points of transition, she is going to experience a struggle internally, and maybe even externally, about what she knows to be true of her own experience and how that directly contradicts what is expected of her. These expectations can come from others, from the big and overwhelming influence of society or culture, or even from you. These expectations can be about sitting still and behaving in a "ladylike" way, taking sewing class instead of auto-shop, not saying something if it creates conflict, or pretending to not know the answer to make a boy feel smarter. You have the ability to tell her, right from when she's young, that she has the right to do or say anything she wants, as long as it's not hurting herself, or anyone else. She doesn't have to be anyone else's version of her, just to make them comfortable, but she has something unique to offer the world and that the world is missing out if she is just a carbon copy of everyone else. Then, when she approaches puberty, you can anticipate and notice the change in her that begins to take place, and fight for opportunities for her to be her *real* self. You can make home a safe place for her to truly be herself, so that no matter what happens out in the world, she knows there is always a relationship (with you), a place (at home) when she is totally completely enough, just as she is. You can help her become aware of that transition as it happens, to slow or eradicate the silencing of herself. And, you can prepare her to deal with the backlash that happens when other people get uncomfortable. By doing this, you prevent her from experiencing the inner turmoil that comes from knowing she is accepted but only if she is who someone else wants her to be. This inner turmoil can be at the root of anxiety, depression, eating disorders, and so many other issues that we struggle with silently as women. Most of all, when you love her as she is, and she loves herself as she is, she knows that giving herself up for the sake of others just isn't worth it. Here's the most difficult part: you can also help her learn how to balance the things that are true for her, with what is valuable to her—keeping her relationships authentic, and close. This is that tricky balance of self in relationship.

MENTAL FREEDOM

Being able to teach her how to do these things is a byproduct of us being able to think critically about the world we are in. This leads us back to the idea of mental freedom, which Dr. Piran identified as one of the three pillars of being able to experience embodiment—a radical self-love. Mental freedom can only come out of being able to assess and think analytically about what's going on around us without the worry of what that will cost us. The image that comes to mind when I think about the relationship between critical thinking and mental freedom is of a person exploring off a beaten path. When we're used to taking the well-worn trail, the work has been done for us. But to see things most people don't see means venturing into the uncertainty, using our discernment to figure out the placement of our feet, with no guarantees of what we will experience. It may be lonely, or painful, at times—sharp twigs scratching our calves, or the accidental step into an unseen puddle—but there is freedom with going a different way, and in that the excitement of being fully alive.

Critical thinking relates directly to what I wrote about in the chapter on media. If we're passively consuming ideas, like the ones communicated in the media, whether they're subtle and sneaky, or overt and obvious, we're not actually free. We're stuck in a system that has power over us. Some of the ideas that help girls think critically to achieve mental freedom related to embodiment include being aware of objectification. As mentioned in an earlier chapter, objectification occurs when girls and women are seen as objects, just bodies, particularly for the enjoyment or pleasure of others.[33] Self-objectification occurs when we start to internalize these ideas, and play along. This can look like doing things to our bodies (certain exercises, taking medications, dieting in certain ways) to make the object of our body look more pleasing and desirable to others, but take away from our experience as a self. Doing this almost always leads to thinking about our bodies in a way that makes us preoccupied with our appearance, and how others see us. Remember what you read earlier about being what someone wants you to be? That happens in all parts of our lives as women, not just in how we share our thoughts and ideas, or not, but also in how we expect ourselves to look. The body and the mind together, after all, make up who we are.

MENTAL FREEDOM AND IDENTITY

Mental freedom is our ability to explore who we are. Instead of feeling like what is expected of us is so hardwired into us that we forget there is any other way of being, we are the ones who are determining who we get to be. This means that we might not belong to a specific social group. I might really want to fit in with the "artists" or the "cheerleaders," but I might be pretending to be someone I am not so that I can fit in. And realizing that I want to be myself instead of pretending might mean that I'm fully me, but don't fit in anywhere. That can be painful, but it doesn't mean we are any less valuable. When working towards mental freedom, it can be important to ask ourselves questions like, what are the things that are expected of me? What are the shoulds in my life and where did I learn those? Does it have to be that way? What do I like about it, and what makes it hard for me to be healthy as a woman? As yourself how many of the things you expect of yourself you learned from your mother, and the other women in your life. If you're a mother, notice if the things you're asking of her are actually just reflections of what you want for yourself. I think here of the classic example of the mother who was a cheerleader in high school, and wants her daughter to do the same so they can have that shared experience together. However, wanting your daughter to belong to that group is more about you then it is about her. So, although you are encouraging her and supporting her to be active, doing it in a way that doesn't allow her to decide what's important to her may be experienced by her as being more restrictive than anything. Maybe that was what happened for you growing up—your mother tried to live out her dreams through you.

The cost of thinking for yourself, exercising your mental freedom, means that figuring out what you want might be different from what others want for you. This might rub up against other people's expectations. It can create challenges and put some of our needs in conflict—when belonging is just as important as thinking freely, it can be hard to meet both needs at the same time when other people don't like when our own ideas differ from theirs. We can be tempted to satisfy our relational longings, our desire to connect, but in doing so deny the parts of us that make us who we really are. It can sometimes be easier as an adult than as a kid to exercise mental freedom and then to find a group of like-minded people. But it can still be difficult if we don't fit into a narrowly defined group. If this feels scary, or you have a daughter for whom this would be scary, think of rehearsing the following pep talk with her, or with yourself: *Sometimes it feels really good to be a part of something, but I don't have to be someone I am NOT in order to try and earn that belonging. It's always good to be kind and respectful to other people, because we all deserve kindness and respect. But I don't have to agree with everyone just to feel like I deserve to belong. Maybe right now there aren't (a lot of) people around me that I know of who I feel really understand me, but if I look, they will be out there, and when I find them I will be so glad that I can be me, who I really am, not just the person everyone has wanted me to be.*

It's important for us to know that we cannot please everyone, we are not meant to be liked by everyone, and that there are groups that we don't have to fit into. And that is ok. In fact, the more we know ourselves, love ourselves, as we are, the more that not being part of that group will feel like a manageable discomfort, instead of social suicide. When this is really hard, it is especially important to find activities, groups, networks, where connecting with others is where we can be "as we are."

CHALLENGING IDEAS OF FEMININITY

Mental freedom also means being able to interact with ideas of womanhood and femininity in a way that challenge conventions that are outdated and oppressive. What I mean by this is that there are stories that in Western culture we are told about being a woman, that give us a clear box to be in, an easy target to shoot for, but are not necessarily psychologically, socially, or spiritually healthy, and limit the fullness of the experiences we can have as humans. Part of having mental freedom means examining these ideas (the shoulds for women) and thinking more about whose ideas these are. When women dare to live a fuller life as a woman than the narrow confines of the "box of femininity," we know that this can be liberating and fulfilling, giving us freedom to think differently about ourselves, about what makes us beautiful, and what we can say and do in our lives. Think about all the things you were ever told about being feminine, about being a woman, about being a girl. What about all the things that were never said. Think about the first times you heard that girls are "sugar and spice, and everything nice" but don't play hockey, sweat, wear comfortable clothes, or cut their hair short. These narrow ideas about what it means to be a woman are actually proven to be related to self-hatred, eating disorders, and a number of other really difficult mental health issues. Think about how those archaic ideas might actually have limited all of the things you could have experienced in life, and what and who you might be if you never had those closing in around you. I can just imagine some of you with this book in your hands, trying to visualize yourself in a full football uniform, and feeling the awkwardness and almost sinfulness in the unfemininity of it. Or maybe some of you feel like you took your first deep breath of freedom in twenty years. Have these conversations with yourself and the women around you, and listen to yourself, and each other. In really listening we are liberating ourselves from the silence and constriction of this feminine box, and reminding ourselves that our thoughts and feelings do matter, even when they are counter-cultural. Maybe especially when they are counter-cultural.

The thing that gets me excited about this all is when I get to see the proof that doing this actually helps girls and women be healthy. The relationship between mental freedom and embodiment goes both ways: girls who are more mentally free are able to be more embodied, and girls who are more embodied are better able to resist the harmful ideas of femininity that limit who they are.[34] Girls who were embodied were able to reject, not just in their heads, but out loud in words, the narrow definitions of what it means to be a girl, in a way that liberated them. Although it is sometimes a dirty word, feminist approaches to critically thinking about the world fit the bill quite nicely here. There is research to support the positive relationship between feminist idea, and healthy attitudes towards one's body.[35] And, because we're all relational, think about how empowering it would be to know that—on the dance floor, at volleyball practice, in the food court, whatever—you or your girl were so mentally free and satisfied "as is" that it changed the way that other girls and women saw themselves. There will always be the women who are envious of others' freedom, but you do not have to "play small" to protect them from the pain of their own desire to be more free. We are usually more familiar with a "negative spiral" or "catastrophic snowball" where things feel like they feed off each other, just getting worse and worse. I always like to remind my clients that there is such a thing as a positive spiral (not just a negative spiral)—change and freedom can start in small ways, and can lead to bigger and more important victories. This is especially true when we consider the work of Jean Baker Miller—that as relational beings we have the power to add more to each other's lives, and in doing so become more of ourselves.

SOCIAL POWER

If we start to think critically about our culture, and examine objectification, we can see that if having a body that looks a certain way makes us valued as women, that appearance is often directly related to our social power. Social power is the third pillar addressed by Dr. Piran as a contributing factor to embodiment. The inverse is also true: social oppression can limit the feelings of safety and goodness in being us. Social power is the experiences we have in life which privilege us to be connected to others who we consider important to us, and be treated equitably. Having social power means we are less likely to experience oppression and victimization, but if we do, we can stand up against unfair treatment of ourselves and others. Again, this relates back to the idea of voice and critical thinking. If we don't really see what's wrong, because we are working so hard to fit in that we go along with the social tide, we can lose our ability to speak up, to have a voice for ourselves and others. This can create added layers of pain for us if we feel unable to speak against the unfair treatment of ourselves. The most interesting analysis I ever heard of eating disorders, and what's going on for the woman who's struggling with disordered eating, is that eating disorders can be about trying to restore social power.[36] This disorder is vanity, but about a woman who is wanting to be accepted and valued by others, so she is trying to change her size in order to get those things she so desperately longs for: the acceptance and validation that culture promises if only we look a certain way. But, in doing so, the disorder takes over and she somehow gets stuck in the loop, always chasing something— losing five more pounds—in order to make herself feel what she's always wanted herself to feel. Like eating disorders, our relationships with our bodies as women are a reflection of our social context. If we were living in a culture where big was beautiful, then instead of trying to lose weight, or diet endlessly, our young girls would be trying to pack on the pounds in order to be desired and feel like they belong. Having been born with a certain body, or within a certain social or economic class, can come with privilege that gives a girl more power—like having unique and attractive physical traits, such as big blue eyes, or long lean legs. Having a certain appearance can give us more certain social power because it protects from the opposite—social disempowerment, like teasing, being ostracized, and feeling as if you don't belong. For this reason it makes it important that we have people in our lives who make us feel less alone, and know us as we really are. Social power is compromised when a person feels as if he or she is less valuable or human, or is made to feel like a minority by others even when this isn't necessarily the case. No one deserves this, ever. And when it happens, it affects our experiences of ourselves, in all ways.

Even in a book talking about body image, it would be negligent to talk about social power and the devaluation of people without talking about race. More so than many other observable qualities about a person, race has been used throughout history as a tool of oppression. In a conversation about social power, as it relates to a woman's experience of embodiment, race plays a significant factor in what women are taught to believe about their bodies. As I have written previously, what we are told about and experience through our bodies is closely tied to our experiences of 'self.' The research that links social power to embodiment, and social devaluation to disembodiment, means that minority girls and women can face additional barriers when fighting to love their bodies compared to those who don't also experience racial oppression. It's complicated, and as a white woman I can only speak about this relationship based on what I know from what research in this area tells me. I have so much to learn from women for whom it is a reality to face the challenges of being a woman layered with having their experiences both of insight and oppression diminished, if not silenced all together. There is so much more that we need to learn about this as researchers, clinicians, and humans to end the oppression of all people, especially women of color, so that all of us can be free.

AMBER'S STORY

This is where I want to introduce you to Amber, and her mother Bev. Amber does the concept of "voice" very well, and has even learned to have and love her voice in spite of feeling like it created conflict in her relationship with her friends and with her mother at times. Amber's story also tells us about the normal struggle to balance the individual self and the relational self, and how she, as a new young mother, has struggled to remain mentally free, in spite of all the scripts about mothering, being a woman, and having a daughter telling her she should do and be.

When Amber talks about her body, she is lively and animated. She has bright red hair—like fire on her head, like a metaphor for the spark and aliveness that she carries inside. When she told me about growing up, she told me that she remembers it being a time free of adult concerns, and getting just to focus on "kid stuff." This changed around puberty when she started to notice her body in a new way, particularly how it was similar, or different, to the other bodies around her. This was most difficult when her friends were developing quicker than she was, which made her feel different than them, especially when other people noticed the differences between her and them and pointed it out to her. In listening to Amber talk about her story what I found was most powerful was that in it all, she managed to retain her voice, right at the time when most girls would start to lose their knowing, and begin to silence themselves. In a demonstration of this, she told me about a time when she tried to speak truthful and kind words to her friends about their appearances, but because her body was more slender and petite than theirs, she was shamed, learning quickly that as women, the only way we're "supposed" to relate to each other is to put ourselves down. We learn that something kind and reassuring about ourselves or about others, especially when people are envious of us, is wrong. When another woman tells you that she hates her thighs, and you tell her that you think they are beautiful and womanly, and that in fact you like your thighs the way they are, it is like you have all of a sudden become the enemy. In that moment with her peers, because she was speaking well of her body and others' bodies, her opinion didn't matter. Amber's slow-to-develop body didn't look like others so her opinion about bodies didn't matter to her friends. The irony here is that even though Amber's slender body was perhaps more stereotypically ideal, it didn't make her accepted by others and loved; it almost did the opposite. Her prepubescent body made her unsafe, a threat, to the other girls who were struggling with their insecurities.

When Amber told me about this experience, she started to cry. It was obvious that in spite of the experience being well over a decade ago, feeling the tension between wanting to belong, and being excluded over something she had no control of, still felt painful. She recalls being around thirteen years old, and at a friend's house in the backyard by the pool, and one of her friends was inside because she wasn't feeling comfortable with her body. Her friend said that she "felt fat" and Amber tried to tell her she wasn't, and she looked great. When she said this, Amber's friend told her to leave, and that her input wasn't allowed because she was thinner. Back then, it was confusing and upsetting. When she talks about it now her ability to think critically about the situation shines through. She says, "I didn't feel like I was allowed to participate, that maybe, I wasn't enough. You know, the goal of people in our culture is to be thin, and to be this, and to be that. I still felt like [what happened] wasn't ok ... like it's not actually ok to be that way either, because of the way it affects your relationship with people. Do you know what I mean?" I did, and still do. In her analysis of that experience when she was thirteen, Amber demonstrates her critical thinking, social power (and disempowerment, really), and voice. She was able to shrewdly identify that there is this goal we have as women to be thin, and look a certain way. But, if we happen to arrive there, it's still not enough to make us happy because it cuts us off from other people. And, being connected to people is part of what makes us feel alive and fulfilled. Amber also saw how her image alone disconnected her from others, not by her own choice, but because it was threatening to the other girls who wanted to have a body that looked like hers. She tried to stand up to her friend, in a way that was supposed to make her friend feel better, but it actually just pushed her away. This is a special example of how speaking the truth can make others uncomfortable, even if the truth we're telling them is something that could help them heal. They might not be ready to heal, creating tension in the relationship. Amber addresses just how challenging that tension was, between wanting to stand up to her friend and speak the truth, wanting to be accepted for who she was, not shunned. She realized that in that moment she couldn't have them both. She later identified something crucial to how we often relate to each other as girls and women—I remember this a lot while going through puberty, and hear it in lots of older women going through menopause: commiserating with other girls or women about how much we dislike our appearance is something that brings us together with them. Or at least, it makes us feel like we're in the trenches together, as equals. The academic term for this is "fat talk," a term coined by Mimi Nichter, and it is how women feel like they bond by sharing their stories of body hatred. Amber says, "If you're good friends with someone, and you think that you are fat, and she thinks that she's fat, then you both think that you are fat, and you're comfortable with each other, because you're uncomfortable with yourself, and she's uncomfortable with herself. But if there is someone who is uncomfortable with themselves, and you're comfortable with yourself, especially if it's really obvious that you're either of those things, it's awkward, it just doesn't make space for that." What Amber describes is that intersection of our body-shame and our desire to be relational. When we dislike our bodies, and we know that other women do too, we can feel connected to each other because of it. But, if we feel differently about our bodies, because our bodies are such a central part of who we are in this world, that felt difference can feel like an enormous emotional gulf, apparently wide enough to sever a connection. Thinking about this part of Amber's story makes me wonder how things could have been any different. What would have happened if Amber knew that being excluded was more about the other girls' shame than her inability to belong? Or, what if Amber spoke to that girl in a way that preserved the connection, but also told the truth? It gets me thinking about what that would sound like, and how you might be able to speak up, be yourself, but also stay connected to others. In the short game, as in that specific moment when Amber spoke to her friend, maybe connection needs to take a back seat to standing up to injustice or untruth, so that in the long run, as women we can create relationship built on self-love and mutual respect, not just joining in to tearing ourselves and others down.

Amber was eventually able to find satisfying relationships with other women who were respectful towards herself and the others. She talks about these women in a way that highlights that they have something really special. Having met in high school and still friends, instead of having to be mutually hating of themselves to connect, they all feel really built up by each other. These other women are also confident, and she believes that having them in her life added depth to the way she saw the world. Through connection with these other women she says that she has been able to experience even more mental freedom. They were authentic and honest together, but in a way which helped them each be able to think more critically about the world. About these friendships she says, "There is life in those conversations, and life in our friendships. We're talking about life-giving things; I feel that makes a huge difference. Like, if we got stuck up on counting calories, all these things that people do, it's not a conversation. So we get to talk about good things, we talk about heart things, things that are really important, things that actually make a difference." In finding these friends, she was able to become more of herself, have a voice, and be connected all at the same time. This relationship sounds like such a contrast from that experience she had at age thirteen by the pool.

After finishing high school, Amber left the country for a unique educational experience, got married, got pregnant shortly after that, and gave birth to a girl. Through describing pregnancy and birth, her unique perspective on her body is hard to miss; she described enjoying watching her body grow and get big. She said that it helped her anticipate motherhood. During the birth, she experienced a new level of her own courage and strength. She described it as painful and challenging, but was surprised at the display of her own ability. Through this she realized more fully than before what she (her mind and body together) were capable of. That is a prime example of physical strength and power, leading to more appreciation and respect for the self *as* the body. She describes it in the following way: "Being pregnant and delivering a baby was un-believe-able. Right away, right after she was out and I had her on me I was like, 'I want to do that again.' I just loved it. I loved that I could do that, I love that my body was made to do this, I loved that."

Like puberty all over again, Amber was challenged to accept her body after birth. Having always felt accepting and loving towards herself, she was actually surprised by her feelings towards her body, having anticipated that she would be comfortable with the changes she was to experience. For Amber, it was less about how her body looked, and more about getting used to it feeling different to be in her own skin. Having her body change so rapidly in so many ways, in such a short amount of time, required her to adjust mentally and learn to love herself as she is, even when that is different than what she had known before. Seeing her body be powerful directly affected her ability to accept herself as a new body—that power helped her accept the stretch marks that go along with the life-giving experience of birth, as a badge or marker of her experience of growth and strength. She has also found it helpful to have a husband who has been supportive. He has encouraged her, and reminded her that he loves her for all of who she is, not just how her body looks. It has been a few years now, and Amber is at a place where she has been able to find joy in how her body has changed. To Amber, embracing those changes has allowed her to be more engaged in life, keeping her present, instead of always wishing she was a different version of herself. When speaking about her desire to continue to accept herself as she ages, practicing kindness to herself at all of life's stages, she recognizes that it's not the same for all women.

AMBER AND HER MOTHER

She says sadly about the consequences of her mother's difficulty with accepting herself, "She's missing out, and I don't want to miss out." Amber's own experiences of having and being a female body starkly contrast those of her mother. This is not unlike the other ways that Amber is different from her mother. In their separate interviews they both talk about when Amber was a teenager how they seemed to disagree endlessly about almost everything. That sounds difficult, but also typical of a teenage girl, especially one who is trying to figure out who she is, and push against her mother. Through finding her own voice, Amber has been able to create an experience of being her own self. She seems to have found freedom in ways that her mother hasn't yet been able to. Amber talks about knowing how dissatisfied her mom is with her own body, and how this comes out in subtle comments about herself as she ages, or other people's appearances. Bev has mentioned, off the cuff on a number of occasions, how unhappy she is with her body after having several children. To which Amber responded (watch for social power and mental freedom here): "No, Mom, you've had five kids, it's not going to be the same, and its shouldn't be the same, and that's ok." This statement reminds me of the idea of the ladder discussed in the first chapter, Amber has gone up high, and is reaching down a hand to her mother, saying, "Mom, come up, it's great up here."

As with most of the mothers and daughters I interviewed, there was a lot of silence between Amber and Bev about menstruation, puberty, and sex. Bev did speak up timidly once—that Amber can recall—to talk about periods. Several times in each of their interviews, they both mentioned how outspoken Amber was, and is. And how that has actually been something Amber has used to connect with and build her mother up. She took her mother bathing suit shopping, and after much back and forth, convinced her mother to get a stylish bikini for an upcoming vacation. That reminded me of the way Amber advocated for her friend in the bikini at thirteen, only this time, it was her mother's confidence she was fighting for. Amber's advocacy for other women is inspiring, reminding the women around her to take pride in their appearance no matter what, creating a sense of connection and safety within and between them. Amber's advocacy for her mother while bathing suit shopping is a great example of Amber having a voice, and standing up against injustice, even if the injustice was internal within her mom's thoughts, or those of her thirteen-year-old friends.

So much of Amber's mental freedom, social power, and voice are revealed in her relationships with others and how she speaks about those relationships. She speaks passionately about setting a positive example for her young daughter, watching the little things she says and does in front of her daughter to make sure what she is communicating is in line with what she wants her daughter to know. One thing she wants her daughter to know is that as girls and women, we don't have to have a culturally defined experience of our body. For Amber, her faith and spirituality is a big part of this. She says when she has unhealthy and destructive thoughts she knows are influenced by the media and culture—thoughts about needing to look or act a certain way—she challenges those thoughts by seeing how they measure up to what she knows to be true about herself spiritually. She describes the refining process of her faith, and how she has sought to see beauty in the way God sees beauty, not in the way our culture sees beauty. This has translated into how she wants to be a positive role model for her daughter. Since becoming a mom she has started to hear the conversations her mother, and mother in-law, have in a new light. Although it has been difficult, she has decided to speak up, using her voice to act on behalf of her daughter, asking her family members to pay attention to what kinds of things they say around the "little ears." In a recent conversation with one family member, she told them what she wanted to protect her daughter from. In doing so she faced the uncomfortable reality that speaking up might actually create tension in the relationship, but chose to do so anyway in order to shield her daughter. Before this, the conversation among these family members seemed to always focus on weight, dieting, and how to look more beautiful. Amber says, "In the two and a half, or three years since I've met [her], I've had more body conversations than ever in my whole life. ... I decided I would say something because of my girl. ... Me and my husband are very aware of this, but we're not the only places she's going to learn these things from; she's going to learn these things from [family members]." By speaking up, she is not only acting on behalf of her own daughter, but on behalf of herself, her family members, and all girls and women everywhere—working against the narrow definitions of beauty and femininity that silence and disempower women. Amber is not waiting for her daughter to grow up to start being aware of the dialogues that are going on, or to start talking directly to her daughter about bodies. She is working, even now, to make sure that what she communicates through actions and words send a very clear message that our bodies as women are just one part of who we are: our bodies are good. We can celebrate, respect, and care for our bodies, even if they look different than the bodies of women in media, or bodies of women around us.

BEV, AMBER'S MOM

In doing this research, my supervisor and I knew we were looking for young women who love themselves as they are, but were not expecting to find that this was not necessarily the case for their mothers. This dynamic is true of Amber's and Bev's relationship. Bev, Amber's mother, is the mother of five, and has a very complex relationship with her body. She was very thin when she was younger, and was teased as a result. She tells me that being teased in this way made her feel helpless and insecure at the time, but she told me that thinking about it later made her think that she had actually been quite fortunate to be so thin growing up, because she believes it wasn't as difficult socially as it could have been had she been larger. Although it's been at least four decades since this happened, she remembers being a child, wearing her bathing suit, and a friend said to her, "You have one hip bigger than the other." She recalls this being the time when she first started to notice her body in a new way, in a more objectified and critical way. This hypercritical and objectified awareness of her body is the way she relates to herself, even still. She remembers desiring larger breasts sometime in her thirties, but stops the story to say to me, "Don't we all"? In her question, she asks me to join with her in normalizing her dissatisfaction with her female body, and without meaning to, points to the cultural script most women carry to be unsatisfied with how their body looks and feels, always desiring to have a body that looks more closely in line with the "ideal."

Like the other mothers interviewed, Bev was having a hard time adjusting to her now aging, perimenopausal body. When she told me the story of her relationship with her body-self throughout life, it sounded like she was now mourning the loss of her younger, pre-motherhood body. She told me about learning to accommodate aging by dressing in a way that hid or accented certain parts of her body. But in listening to her tell her story, it sounds like she is feeling a mix of resignation and tentative acceptance with her current body, knowing she can't really change it. She says, "I don't worry about it too much, because it doesn't seem to matter what you do, it's going to be there." This is radically different from the way Amber speaks about hoping to age. Unlike her mother, Amber is hoping instead to value her stretch marks, sagging breasts, and wrinkles as a badge of honor for a life well lived. When I asked Bev to complete the sentence "my body is," she replied by saying, "It's not perfect, but I'll take it," demonstrating again this dissatisfaction mixed with tentative acceptance and resignation. Bev answered my next question "women's bodies are ..." by saying "they're amazing, just the way they work ... and all they go through, and produce life, and it's flabbergasting how wonderful they are...." Can you see the difference between those two statements, how she sees herself, and how she sees other women? When she says this I'm struck with a mix of confusion, joy, and disbelief. In listening to her, she's saying the "right thing," the thing that this study is all about—women loving their bodies. But I can't help but wonder if that is Bev doing what we all struggle with as women—saying what someone else wants to hear, instead of how we really feel. I wonder about this because of how different her two answers are—she describes her body like a broken down old piece of machinery, on its last legs, but when she is talking about women in general, somehow our bodies are miraculous and beautiful. Or maybe she really does believe it, that her relationship with her body is a painful one, and somehow she is the exclusion from the general sacredness and beauty of women. I do this, I hear lots of people do this, in so many areas of our lives: "They are amazing, just as they are, but I need to be perfect in order to be "good enough." It makes me sad thinking about this, wishing for her, and all the other women out there who feel or think in this way, that somehow these two different answers would align—that we would be able to feel about our own bodies the way that we feel about women's bodies in general.

As we continued the interview, I kept getting glimpses of deeper awareness taking root in Bev. I was wondering if this was because of the questions themselves, and our conversation. She said a few times how hard the questions were for her to answer, because she doesn't often think about herself, her body image, embodiment. Bev suspected that this "not thinking about her body" was probably a result of being so busy, with five children, and having little time to reflect. My guess is that this is like most women in our culture: we are both rarely thinking about ourselves, and always thinking about ourselves. Maybe the distinction is that when we think about ourselves, our bodies, our appearance, our thoughts are critical or shaming, maybe even objectifying, but we probably don't take time to intentionally sit with our thoughts about our bodies and appearance, noticing them, naming them, thinking critically about where they come from.

"DROOBIES"

Ironically, not reflecting and talking about our bodies was something she described her own mother doing, which really bothered her. Bev's mother also had five children, and she recalls that her mother never took time to speak with her about deeper issues, like the ones we were talking about in the interview. "My mother was in a different generation," she said. "There wasn't a whole lot of open dialogue about anything." She remembers approaching her mother about these things at times, only to have her mother switch topics and laugh the subject off dismissively. After growing up into her own woman, she is now able to understand this as her mother's inability to communicate openly, but remembers that at the time this left her feeling unprepared for her journey to become a woman and feeling quite alone. Because of all of this, she wanted to do better for her children, and be more emotionally available for them than her mother was for her. She speaks to how difficult this actually was, reflected on worrying at times that she could have done a better job of speaking up, seeing how similar she has become to her own mother in many ways. This is one of the most notable differences between Amber and Bev— as Amber has always been vocal and opinionated. Bev reflected on how this made Amber one of the most difficult children to parent, but that it seems all worth it now because of the free and confident woman Amber has become today. It is clear as Bev talks that the disagreeing and arguing that was a big part of Amber finding her voice was challenging at the time, but Amber is very much her own person, and Bev loves that about her. Amber was able to push back and challenge her mother's opinions and ideas, in a way that actually helped Amber learn to find her voice. And, because of the safety and security of her parents' love, she found a way to think for herself. The part of the story that feels most satisfying to me as an interviewer, therapist, researcher is that Amber's mental freedom and voice may have created conflict at first that jeopardized the relationship, but we can see now how it has come full circle. Not only has Amber become her own person, but her tenacity and rejection of cultural norms of beauty and femininity have allowed her to advocate on her mother's behalf as well. Now she is able to be in a relationship with her mother in a way that has helped her mother experience more freedom and embodiment that she would not know if she did not have Amber to learn from, and grow with. Amber's rare perspective on women's bodies allows her to find joy in things that typically cause women fear, like birth, aging, and a changing body. I'll let Amber say this in her own words: "I know my mom is [dissatisfied with her body]; I don't want to be dissatisfied. I want to enjoy myself, I want to enjoy my life. I want to allow my husband to enjoy me, and if I don't feel comfortable, then I'm not there. You know, I just can be, and I want to be, I want to be comfortable being naked with him, that is so important through our whole life, like whatever stage I go through. If I'm uncomfortable, then [our relationship] becomes uncomfortable. I see that there, it makes me more aware of things, like how [comfort and discomfort in our bodies] affect other things, right? It's not just me. I really want to embrace age, like growing old. I want my hair to grow grey, I want it to go white actually, I would love that. I want to embrace those things. I want to embrace wrinkles and sags. My husband and I joke about having droobies, like droopy boobs. I want to embrace my droobies, you know? All of those things. I want to age well in my heart. I feel like my mom is missing out, 'cause I know there is something better and she's missing out on that, and I don't want to miss out." My jaw drops whenever I read this. Amber is committed to continuing her story of healthy relationship with herself, in her body, in a way that can be an example to other women, her daughter in particular. Her passion and acceptance are going to make her an incredible mother, and a great example of how we can continue to grow in our relationship with others, and ourselves, through time. To me, I can see the intergenerational piece here so clearly: Amber wanting freedom for her mother, herself, and her daughter. What if we could all feel this way? What if aging, grey hair, and sagging breasts were not swear words? Amber's words are so profound; she acknowledges that her mother's dissatisfaction with her aging body make her miss out on life. Although it is important to acknowledge the grief and pain of change with age, when we are wishing away the present for something we used to have, we can miss what we do have, who we are, now, and the beauty in that.

In the stories of these two women we see clearly that in spite of her mother's own struggle with her body, Amber learned from an early age how to think for herself—even though this meant lots of arguing and disagreement during her teenage years. Because of her ability to have a

146

voice, and stand firm in who she is, she's been able to be critical of the societal scripts around her, of what it means to look and act a certain way as a woman. This has allowed her to stand up for herself, and push back against those ideas, feeling powerful and connected to her voice enough that she is ok with disagreeing with others. This has not limited her ability to be a relational self, and she's found ways to maintain and nurture relationships that matter, and help her feel like she has a place with others where she belongs. Amber's healthy sense of self—having a voice, experiencing social power and mental freedom—is directly related to her ability to love and appreciate herself as a body, regardless of how she looks, changes, performs, moves, and feels.

AGING AS A WOMAN

It seems as though as women in our society age, they disappear. As the script for ideal beauty goes: be thin, sexy, and young. So as women move further and further from the ideal of youth, a few things seem to happen. One option: they work harder than ever before to remain looking and feeling youthful, putting more energy and money into the pursuit of youth the further from it they get. Another option: they work to varying degrees to maintain a feeling and appearance of youthfulness. But they want to appear to age naturally, and put some effort in, while also accepting with some degree of grief the inevitable aging process. Then, there appears to be another group who finds freedom in being further form the societal idea, feeling less pressure than ever before to compete or labor for something that was almost always unattainable, but has become increasingly so. For these women, aging feels like permission to finally not care in the same way that they always did. They finally feel liberated from the expectations on them and their appearance they carried most of their lives, and consequently free from the shame about not being able to meet those expectations. This is an area I'm researching right now as part of my dissertation—it seems that because of aging women's social invisibility (as if culture is saying "if you're not a sex object to us, you have no value"), they are a group of people who are largely underresearched, especially when it comes to their relationships with themselves. Although I wish for all aging women the freedom that some women find in being released from the unrealistic appearance expectations, I long for the day when all women and girls are treated equally, and are recognized as having worth and value regardless of their weight, age, or sex appeal.

FREEDOM AND PROTECTION THROUGH VOICE

In their book *Raising a Daughter*,[37] Jeanne and Don Elium talk about how important it is to help a young girl think for herself. They write, "Betrayal begins early as a mother teaches her daughter how to be sweet, compliant, and silent. ... We fear our daughters' safety if they are too outspoken, too different, too visible" (pg. 134). Although this might come from a protective place, it actually ends up costing your daughter something very precious: herself. They continue on, "When daughters grow up deprived of their 'voices,' something essential is missing. Giving voice to one's thoughts and opinions, fears and triumphs builds self-esteem and courage. Mothers can pass on the lineage of silence and female bondage, or they can empower their daughters to say 'no' to constraints, to argue for their rights, to speak out against injustices, to voice their anger toward violation."[38] What will always be more important than having the right outfit, or the "right body" is finding the freedom and confidence to be ourselves. This is the best gift we can give our daughters, ourselves, and the girls and women around us. If you are a mother, you will likely raise a healthier daughter if she knows how to think for herself, even if this is more frustrating and annoying to you than if she does exactly what everyone says. You can do this by encouraging her to speak up, and by speaking up yourself, talking about your feelings in a productive way, especially when you are hurting, modeling for her how to do the same. The more autonomy and self-determination we have as girls and women, the more protected we will be from things such as body shame, following the crowd, obsessing over thinness, and eating disorder behaviors.[39] Although it might be hard, especially if this has been a struggle for you for a long time, it is never too late to start working on being a more compassionate, accepting, and free version of yourself. It is not too late to dream of a life that is more than being a "good" or "nice" girl, if that means that we silence ourselves, stuff our feelings down, and shut up to make other people comfortable.[40] It may not be popular, and it may feel uncomfortable for you, and for the people who are hearing you, to try out your new voice. So be gracious with yourselves and others in the process.

As you start finding your voice, or figuring out where you left it long ago, you might notice some feelings come up about other women who have "their voice." Pay attention to those feelings, and learn what they tell you about yourself. You might find that in thinking critically about the world, you want others to do the same, or you feel sad that other women don't want to join you in that. You were never meant to play small just to make other people comfortable, and it is possible to be loved and be fully you all at the same time. Although it may not happen without discomfort, returning to your freedom and your voice is a gift you give yourselves, and those around you.

REFLECTION QUESTIONS

- When did you start to experience "loss of voice" or "silencing the self"?
- What was communicated to you about being "good" that has limited your ability to be who you really are?
- What would it be like to be who you really are, if not worried about what other people think?
- Who do you normally hear "fat talk," or who do you normally "fat talk"? Who hears you fat talk? What could you say or do next time to change the direction of the conversation?
- Where do you feel like you most belong?

- What would it "cost" you to speak up where you most needed to?
- Who are you most safe to be your fullest and most free self with? With whom or when do you feel you have to hide yourself?
- When was the last time you sung, like really belted out your favorite song? Try it!

▶ If you have a daughter...
- What messages might you have communicated to your daughter about being "good" that actually serve to limit who she is?
- What might you say next time you see your daughter "stuffing down" her thoughts and feelings?
- What is a good place to start being critical of social and cultural attitudes of femininity?
- Ask your daughter about what her and her friends say about their bodies, weight, image, etc.
- What are some ways that you can value your daughter's opinions, even if you don't agree?
- What are some ways, at home, or with chores, that you can help your daughter feel like she matters?
- Where does your daughter feel like she most belongs? Can you help her find more of these places and people?
- What can you do to help her learn to think critically about how she might have to "give up" parts of herself to fit it?
- When was the last time you just sat and listened to your daughter—learning about who she is and appreciating the way she sees the world?
- Do you normally jump in and correct or criticize, or are you silent and passive, afraid to engage in a dialogue with her?

EIGHT

DEEP AND HIGH: SPIRITUALITY AND THE BIGGER PICTURE

"The wound is where the light enters you."

–RUMI

By the time that things were at their worst with my eating disorder, I had been to several therapists: my mother would tell me that she wanted me to see someone to talk about my eating, and presumably other things. I played along, sometimes. Sometimes I would wait in the waiting room like everyone else, flipping through carefully selected magazines. Then, when it was time for my session, I would put up walls to block the therapists out, hide unconvincingly behind a charade that I hoped would seem angry or tough enough that they wouldn't risk going any further. Even when I was starting to be ready, really ready, to start to begin to heal, I still had to be nudged by my mother—the woman who was fighting painfully for me (and often with me) even when I wouldn't reward her with gratitude or closeness. If I'm more honest, the nudge was really a loving and painful push: my mother almost literally dragging me to a new doctor who specialized in eating disorders, with printed forms that needed to be filled out so I could be admitted to a treatment program. So, because of the nudge-push, I met Liz.

In my first therapy session with Liz, I barely said anything. But it was different this time, I wasn't pushing her away, or pretending, I just didn't know where to begin. When you have been hurting and hiding for so long, simply to let yourself be seen feels hard enough. To invite a stranger behind the walls you have yourself been too afraid to look behind is potentially the bravest and most dangerous thing a person could do. I was ready, which was different, but Liz was different too. Liz was the first therapist I went to who I felt saw me: *me*, not the symptoms of the eating disorder, my spine through my skin, my secrecy, or my defenses. She saw *me*. I was afraid to be seen after all the window shades to my heart had been pulled down for so long, and everything inside felt so chaotic and ugly. It could be argued that other therapists would have done the same if only I had let them, and of course it would have taken me being ready to let them. Maybe it's scary to think of her like every other therapist, because to me she was, and is, a gift of life. Over the course of our work together, having her see *me* became an important part of me healing. And in the safety of our relationship I started to figure out again who I really was. Hating my body, trying to shrink and control my body as a way of running away from pain had become my life, and for a while I forgot that I was anything other than that.

For the first season of our work together, it was like Liz cupped her hands around a barely noticeable flicker within me and protected it from the breeze; she reminded me that there was something within me that was still alive, that never had and never could die. We listened to music, drew, banged on drums sometimes, and breathed deeply together as she helped me remember that I was, that I am, my body (I'm not just a head that is carried around by a vehicle). I can inhabit my body. I am my body. And, she talked, a lot. As a therapist now I don't do with my clients what she did with me, unless I know that for them to just show up is the best thing we could both ask for right now. So either she knew what I needed, or it was meant to be that she was the one to hold my hand on the way out of the pit of death and march tirelessly all the way up. Her talking was like a soothing lullaby for the deepest parts of me, and over time I learned from her how to place my own hands, cupped protectively around the flicker within me that was now a growing flame. I learned to take on the role of balancing gentleness and might to nurture the blaze. When that happened, it was like my mind and my heart opened up, and I started to see and know things I wasn't able to see and know before when I was so shut out from myself and from life. I stopped disappearing—in my body, in my emotions and thoughts. I got really sad, and really angry, and really full of life. I started to think for myself, and learn from other women who were thinking for themselves too. I started to think about what needed to be different for me if I was going to stay alive in the same world that I had gotten sick in.

SOMETHING MORE

There are many people before me who are much smarter than I am,[41] who have identified that when girls and women hate and try and control their bodies, they're actually doing exactly what our culture has told them to do. They are "good" girls and women, existing the very way that the dominant narratives of women and men have instructed them to. But what if culture is wrong? What if, like the women I've described in this book have come to know, the things we are doing as women to earn our "enoughness" in this culture or to feel valuable are empty, actually leading us further away from ourselves, and from what it means to be whole? If that is the case, then we need something more—a new narrative, a different story with which to align ourselves, and a healthier way of knowing our worth. If that's the case, I don't want to be what culture thinks it means to be a "good" woman, or girl, if being good in our culture means having to disappear in our bodies, minds, and thoughts.

Although I never set out looking for it, looking back I am not at all surprised that all of the young women in the study who loved their bodies and themselves had a deep and vibrant spiritual life. When looking for women to participate in this study, I had no idea who would come forward and who would even match the criteria I was looking for, but never thought to ask about spirituality. In their stories each of the women talked about relationships with God, and the earth, desiring connection with other people and living a life that was about more than just "me." They all believed that there is a divine spark within each of us, that to them was a very clear "something more" that made them feel alive, valuable, and not alone in this world, than what our cultural script about femininity and masculinity has to offer. For them, even if the culture said that their body was an object used to bring pleasure to men, or our worth as women is determined by how we look, these women were able to know beyond knowing that they didn't have to subscribe to that. For these women, they believed they were loved and valued, known personally and intimately, by their Creator in a way that transcended their appearance and actually satisfied their deepest longings.

When talking about spirituality, I like C.M. MacKnee's definition: spirituality is defined as a core dimension of humanity that seeks to discover meaning, purpose, and connectedness with self, others, and the ultimate other, also referred to as God, divine Other, or Creator.[42] For some of you, this will make a lot of sense. For others, it may seem like a contradiction to talk about God and being freed from silencing in the same sentence. These stories might be different than yours. Maybe in your life, spirituality was mixed up with religion, and the idea that you could connect with a divine presence in a nonreligious, nonoppressive, nonregulated way is foreign, and God has been associated with suffering. Your experience of spirituality might have been of feeling silenced and oppressed by rules or religion that felt restrictive, or that cause hate and judgment in this world, instead of the connection mentioned in the description above. I was having this conversation with a client in therapy recently, and we used a metaphor of person-to-person relationship to help her reframe her painful past relationship to spirituality: even though we might have been in a painful relationship in the past, maybe even an abusive one, it does not mean that all relationships are bad and abusive. Maybe if we have been hurt by someone badly, then it is scary but healing to be loved by someone else. And, maybe our relationship in the past has been with religion, but not with God, and we have confused the two. So perhaps it will be hard for you to read these women's stories of faith and spirituality without having your own pain be triggered. But I encourage you to read about how their stories are similar to or different from how yours has been, and what a relationship between themselves and ultimate Other, the divine, has opened up for them in their relationship with their bodies, with the fullness of themselves.

KNOWING HER BEAUTY

Several chapters ago I introduced you to Kelsey and the significant shifts she has felt in her relationships to herself and her body. Spirituality is at the heart of those transformations. Her story is still as inspiring to me as it was when I first heard it: she has worked for the love and kindness she feels towards herself. At times, it has been a struggle within her, and that was visible in the way she presented herself to the world. But the shifts towards wholeness, and knowing her value, came from encountering God's love for her in a more profound way. Instead of just knowing God loved her in the way we can know what someone expects of us, like a performance, she *knew* it in a way that she finally believed it to be true: she felt it and let it in, and it reshaped how she saw herself. That is exactly like the definition of spirituality I listed, defined by a relationship and connection. She let the personal and unconditional love of God be what defined her worth, not if she had acne, or if someone else was attracted to her, or if she lost or gained weight. And this was where her freedom came from. Listen again to how she describes this moment where she felt the intersection of her freedom and acceptance of herself, and her encounter with God. "I have a [hormonal condition], so when I'm not on birth control now, I will break out into cystic acne all over my face. I can recall three years ago looking in the mirror and thinking, 'I am so ugly,' because my face would be covered in cystic acne, and I would have to wear so much makeup to cover it up. I had this powerful experience where I was worshipping God, and I was naked, and I had no makeup on, and I looked in the mirror and wrote all over the mirror, in marker, 'I am enough.' I had this realization that my body was connected to who I am, and how I can value myself, or see myself."

As we talked more, she addressed the tension women often feel when they learn that their value is more than their appearance—how can we still acknowledge our beauty, physical and otherwise, without falling into the trap that our beauty, physical and otherwise, defines us? She talks about this tension with lots of people, including her therapist, and says that she now believes that beauty in her, and the world, is a reflection of God, and points us towards our Creator. In short, beauty is an invitation to spirituality. She says that the Creator "made women the pinnacle of creation, women are beautiful, and that beauty can draw people closer to God, so we don't have to think, *"Oh, I can't be beautiful [like our beauty is a distraction], but now that my body image is more positive, I don't think that [God, and body image, and beauty] need to be in opposition to one another. I think that I can still be beautiful, but not let it be my identity, do you know what I mean?"*

It might be useful to pause here for a moment, and reread Kelsey's words. Sit with what she might be communicating, and where it might hit you. When I do that, and let those words sink in, they feel like poetry, philosophy, and scripture all at once, losing me in the complexity of the contradictions and the truth-telling. How can we as women know our beauty, and believe that the divine is revealed in beauty—in us and in the world—without it meaning that beauty is God, or we are God, or it's the most important thing about us? I grew up in the church, and her words go against the stories about women and God that I've always been told:

men are closer to God, and women's beauty is a distraction and therefore must be subdued. I feel the jolt of her experience bumping up against the things I have always been told. Could it be that beauty in all things leads us closer to the divine? Maybe because of the power of beauty, and what it means within the feminine and masculine scripts, we forget what it is pointing us to, and we worship beauty itself: falling into an obsession with one aspect of life that is really just a signpost to something bigger. Maybe beauty is meant to draw us into wonder, and kindness, and honoring the sacredness of life, instead of it being something we live for, or worship, or that turns us or other people into objects that we judge as being more or less valuable than others. And, could it be that maybe beauty means something other than "young" and "thin" and "sexy"? This is where we need something more than our cultural definition to tell us what beauty is, and what role it plays in our feelings about ourselves, and how we relate to each other.

Kelsey goes on to summarize her story, and what has mattered the most: "Although you've seen these shifts, I think that what was consistent was that I felt safe and secure growing up. ... And although there were many bumps in the road, I felt, I feel, like that has served me well. I [was] intentional in addressing these personal issues, and looking internally into myself and into my heart and also looking at God, and I have a loving husband who loves me and encourages me. ... I think for me to have gotten where I am is not without the work and the intention of being aware of the messages that I am being sent, and also the messages I sent, and questioning them." In saying this, she draws the connection between questioning the messages of the world. She believes that in looking to God as her "something more", that unfailing spiritual relationship affirms who she is and her worth as a woman. Later on, when I asked her why she thought she was able to escape eating disorders and body hatred experienced by so many women, she said outright that her faith is a protective factor, that believing she is loved by God is her identity and she believes this is unwavering. As a result, her identity is protected from the messages from culture about women's value coming from a certain look, act, or size. About this she says, "The truest and most pure core of my being is God in me, and I think that's where these messages [about worth] have to come from, and I can't separate myself from them."

There are parts about Kelsey's story that are likely different from yours. Maybe, like me, you read this and yearn to know of or be close to a divine being who loves you as you are, and who invites you into more of yourself, and into having beauty put back in its right place. If the divine is in us, and lives through us, and I believe that that is not just our mind, but our bodies as well, then who we are—all of us—is sacred.

BEING CREATED

Like Kelsey, Carlee spoke about believing that her worth comes from being known and loved by God. It was moving to hear Carlee talk about her beliefs about being created, and what that means about how we treat each other. She expressed that because we are all created and loved by God, we are all equally valuable, and need to treat each other accordingly. I asked her to tell me more about this and she told me what she wants to be able to tell a daughter of hers one day about what it means to be human, and accepting ourselves and how we look, as we are. "This is who you are created to be," she starts off. "When you are created in God's image, why do you want to change who you are?" She identifies that accepting herself comes from believing that she—as she is—is not a mistake. "If you don't [believe in God] maybe that's even more challenging, but for me, I believe we were all created in God's image, and there is no better image to be created in, ever. And there will never be. You need to remember that the person next to you is also created in that image. That person on the street there? Also created in that image. For me that's something I've really started to cling to and say over and over again in the past two years. If we have trouble getting along with someone, or someone is bullying or being bullied, I'm like, 'Who created this person?' It's the same image as who created us all." In saying this, it is like Carlee is literally ripping down the walls that divide us, the pride, social class, race, gender, sexual orientation, education, and that is at the heart of spirituality; the yearning to see the connections among us. This kind of spirituality is political, because it fights against the divides that create power hierarchies, making us feel like one group of people is somehow better than another group of people. Just like beauty can lead us to spirituality, spirituality leads us to equality.

Reading this, and rereading this inspires me. I can remember having this conversation with Carlee doing this interview, and she said it all in such a matter-of-fact way. No overspiritualizing or piousness, just a woman who believes she is lovable, and that is because she was created by God, just like everyone else. Although this is about seeing the divine in other people, it makes other people more human, turning them from objects that we compare ourselves to, or judge, into people with stories, hurts, and longings. She takes this further to say that being unable to let the love of God in gets in the way of really being able to love others. "If you don't love yourself, and if you don't know the [Ultimate Love], I don't think you can really love who we created you to be, and I don't know if you can truly love others the way you are created to love them." We are all connected—that is what I feel laced in these words. It reminds me of Glennon Doyle Melton's phrase "we belong to each other."[43] When we know that, we treat ourselves, and each other, so differently.

THE OTHER PART OF THE GOLDEN RULE

All these themes come up a lot in therapy, as people who are hurting deeply realize they want to be loved, to know they are lovable, to belong. Yet sometimes when we are presented with that love, we realize we are struggling to let it in. But if Carlee's right, not letting love in gets in the way of us really loving others well. If I would have read this several years ago, I might have said it wasn't true: I did not love or like myself much at all, but loving other people was what I did well. I even thought about doing it for a job. But as I got healthier, and stronger, and gave myself more time to see what happened when I started to love myself, I realized I had more to give to other people. I could love them better, deeper, and there was more of me that was alive to love with. I also don't think that loving people well means having fun all the time, and sometimes it means sitting very close to someone in silence when they are grieving, or feeling their own pain, and reminding them that they are not alone. So, the more I loved myself, the more I realized how important it was to continue to work through the hurt I was carrying around. As I did that, it wasn't so scary to sit with other people when they were confronting their pain, because pain wasn't as scary anymore.

For a lot of the mothers I work with in therapy, they want so badly to help their daughters know they are loved and beautiful—but they forget that the same things that make their daughters loved and beautiful are also true about them. As Carlee and Kelsey would say, it's the image of the divine, it's the divine spark, it's being loved by the ultimate source of Love and Life. This is a kind of "golden rule" but in reverse. We normally think of the "golden rule" to mean that because we naturally treat ourselves well, we should treat others just as well. But it works the other way too—if we're used to seeing beauty, goodness, and value in others, and treating them well as a result, we must learn to also treat ourselves the same way. I do not believe that there is anything so wrong, broken, or unattractive about you that you are not worth receiving the kindness you would give others. I can see in Carlee's story a countercultural song: as women we are so often told that we need to take care of everyone else but ourselves, and if ever ourselves, then everyone else first. It's important to be loving and kind to others, but if we are made like them, then we cannot forget that loving others well also means loving ourselves. This might be something you have heard, or been told—an idea that you flirt with but are unsure how to live out. It could be revolutionary for you to show up in your own life, in a way that allowed you to share space with other people, where no one is more important than the other.

CREATIVITY AND PROTECTION

Amber's eyes looked so alive when she was talking about our bodies as women, I could have talked to her for hours about it. Almost speechless, she did her best to summon the appropriate description for how diverse and wildly unique we all are as women. "I just ... they are just ... I love that we are all different." The difference that some of us are so scared of, the ridicule (both internal and external) we can face when we do not measure up to an illusion of perfection, was something that Amber seemed to care nothing for: the differences in how we all love, our shapes and sizes as women, that is what captivated her. If looking differently wasn't so scary, it would make sense that she would have more comfort in her body, no matter what it looked like. The differences in our appearance are a reflection of our uniqueness, and the creativity of our Creator. She says, "I love that beauty can be expressed in so many ways, like visibly in so many different ways, and I love that, it just screams of a creative God. It's just, I love it." This is so different than what we are used to hearing through the media, and believing about ourselves and our bodies: be the same, be young, don't take up space, be thin. But Amber speaks against that plot line, reminding us that how we are unlike others, our uniqueness, is part of how things are supposed to be. It's not a mistake that you and I look different than each other. In other words, it's not a mistake that you are who you are. We are not all supposed to be the same.

Think about how this could change the way we interact with both ourselves and others. Think about what this could mean for how you raise a daughter, and what you teach her about how she looks. Think about how this could help *you* if you realize your daughter, and the other women around you, do not look like the magazines tell us we are supposed to. And, how you knowing all this could help them know it too. What if every time you or another woman in your life said "I don't look like the women on TV, or in the magazines" you truly thought, "Good"? What if every time you looked in the mirror and realized you didn't look like women on TV, or you delighted in your uniqueness? What if not looking like other women was an afterthought, because being different is part of being human and looks are no longer how we need to measure ourselves as women?

Amber believes that measuring our worth by our physical appearance, and how our bodies compare to the bodies of other women, especially the bodies of women in the media, will never fulfill us like we are led to believe. But, it makes sense, she says. "It makes sense that our culture struggles with image because, of course, they don't know God." After saying this she caught herself, and reminded us both that people who have faith or spiritual practices are not automatically inoculated against lies about our bodies. But she hints at there being something about having a relationship of love and life with the divine, a spiritual life, that creates a passionate spark of aliveness in us which is different than simply following a set of rules.

MEET JAYA

When Jaya and I sat down for our interview we were both wrapped in blankets, sitting with big cups of tea on our laps, sitting near the basement windows of her mom's house looking out onto the ocean. I had driven around for a while trying to find the house, and felt rushed and nervous, but as soon as I sat down with her it was like all parts of me settled into their right places. Together, with her, something felt still, in a sacred way. When Jaya speaks about herself it is with confidence and humility. It becomes obvious very quickly when listening to Jaya that she is secure in who she is, yet full of grace and far from conceited. She has eyes that are kind, but piercing, and curly hair that seems to go on and on. And when I asked her, she told me that her name "Jaya" means victory.

Having met in her mother's home for the interview, she was able to get up a few times to grab endearing and hilariously adorable school photos of herself to add to the story of her relationship with her body over time. She showed me a picture of a particularly embarrassing haircut which she believes her hairdresser tricked her into getting by describing it as a "lioness do," but what was really a glorified mullet. We laughed together until it hurt, delighting in the particularly unique and dated hairstyle, and she shone from inside out as she told me that her mother, even to this day, tells her that she thinks that her lioness hairdo is magnificent, never embarrassed, and never inciting shame.

Like the other women I have already introduced, Jaya too feels that her relationship with God—and believing that God lives inside of her—is how she has come to have a healthy and loving relationship with herself as a body. She says, "My body is a temple of God. It is beautiful, it is lovely, it is not accepted and loved by everybody, but it is just right." We do not all have to agree that there is a divine energy, a piece of something/someone sacred dwelling in our bodies, but I imagine that if we lived as if this were true, it could change everything. If we treated our bodies like they are the house of the divine, and that all of the power and love in the Universe *wanted* to live inside of us—*just as we are*—and we didn't have to become "perfect" first, imagine what would be different. Maybe we wouldn't constantly try and numb our feelings by putting too much or not enough food into ourselves. Maybe we would slow down more, instead of beating our body into submission and forcing ourselves to work beyond capacity. Some of us might exercise more, and some of us might exercise less. And, we might all stop regularly to just pause, inhale, and feel how lucky we are to be alive, in that moment, with something sacred within us, and a connection to the rest of the sacredness all around us.

When reflecting on her relationship with God as we were talking about her relationship with her body, she told me about the connections she saw between God's love and her mother's love. A decade ago she was speaking at a youth conference, telling the story about how she had left home at a young age, and when she wanted to come back she said her mom just "dropped everything and took me in without a thought." She said what her mom did finally hit her emotionally as she was speaking on stage. In that moment she says it was like she "got it," finally. After really understanding her mother's love and sacrifice for her in a new way she described how it changed their relationship moving forward. "I just got it. ... I was crying, and it was a pretty neat moment. I'm so very, very thankful for my mom, and ever since then it's been nothing but further depths of richness." When I listened to Jaya describe her relationship with her mom, it reminded me of the way the other women spoke about God: profound and limitless love. There was nothing she could do or not do to stop her mother from loving her, and the understanding that love came after the fact. I imagine that the story between Jaya and her mother is one that most of us share with our mothers and/or daughters: as daughters we never know the great sacrifices and gifts of love our mothers have made for us, often until much later than when they were most obvious. Or, we take for granted the small, simple things that our mothers have always done, and probably always should do, as they care for us. Even if it is what they should do, it is no less an act of love. As mothers, your daughters may not have the eyes to see the way you love them, and at times it might break your heart into a thousand pieces. They may even confuse your love with trying to stifle or control them. In my understanding of the complexity of the mother-daughter relationship, those can both be true: that you were loving and they felt stifled. But, I imagine in time they will be able to see what you did as the best way you knew how to love at the time. And in time, you will be able to see how you might have gotten in the way, and say you're sorry.

Just by listening to her talk, with wisdom and reflectivity of someone three times her age, I can feel her rootedness in the things that she believes. She says that because of what she has learned, and her role in the lives of many young women, she has a responsibility to connect with the things she does, to make sure the messages she sends other women are congruent with what she wants to model for them. In learning how to be in a relationship with her Creator she says, "It's been a huge teacher for me about how I connect with things like food, and how I look at myself in the mirror, and how I exercise, and how I talk with people. ... I have confidence that my image is secure, and that is massive. I don't have to try and seek the approval of [men] or women." Knowing her worth, through being loved by God and her mother, helped Jaya step outside the judgment of other people, bringing her into more freedom.

I think mothers have the important task of loving their daughters tirelessly, even when it hurts, showing them always that their worth does not come from any one part of them, especially not their bodies, size, appearance, perceived attractiveness, or conformity to feminine gender scripts. An important job for mothers is showing their daughters what it means to be a heathy (I did not choose the word "perfect" on purpose) woman, and do their best to reflect how God sees us, as described by the women I interviewed, that they are valuable, sacred, unique, beautiful, and not alone. Mothers have the difficult task of pouring love into their daughters right from the beginning of life, to help them know they are loved—insulating them the way that God's love insulated Jaya, reminding her that no matter what anyone else says she knows she is loved. This love is protective against the harmful experiences we can have in the world, and can shape a sense of self from early on that is secure and rich with self-kindness.[44]

Love, both from mothers (and fathers) and from God, is powerfully protective against the oppressive and silencing cultural messaging about being a girl or a woman. Although there is proof in these women's stories, the research conducted for this book, there is lots of other evidence that spirituality and faith practices can be protective for girls and women. The researchers, clinicians, and theorists which make up the APA's task force on the Sexualization of Girls and Women[45] remind us that spiritual and faith practices are protective against sexualization, and can give us other ways of thinking about ourselves and each other as girls and women.

Jaya says that she knows she is a lucky one to be able to love her body in a world where most women don't. "I've been plucked and chosen and I don't deserve it; I don't know why I've been chosen to be like this. I know that God has very clearly protected me and given me a good mother to love me and show me that beauty does not just consist of [how our body looks]." Even in her teenage years when she wasn't as close to her mother, she believes that her Creator's love for her was evident through her friends to help her learn that our bodies are not our only source of worth, and that we can still be beautiful but know that we are not defined by beauty. This friend, Jaya said, consistently showed her that what our body looks like isn't what makes us valuable, and that no matter what she looked like, she was and is beautiful. Thinking about the spiritual dimension to our lives might make you feel uncomfortable. Others of you while reading this will feel curious, or alive. It's hard to ignore this theme running through each story in far more ways than I could ever recount in this book. And, it would actually be unethical in my research to ignore a prominent theme that showed up repeatedly. But like Jaya, Kelsey has no other way to explain why she—unlike so many other women—is a young adult woman with a healthy body image, and loving relationship with all parts of herself. Her only way to explain this is that it was a miracle. She told me the story of when she was a child and an older woman, a spiritual elder in her community, spoke a protective, spiritual bubble around her when she was a child in the form of prayer. She credits this as making the difference in her life. Without this, she believes her relationship with her body may have turned out very differently. She says, "There is something in terms of resilience or spiritual protection that protected me from going down a [road] that would have been unhealthy or hurtful to me." To Kelsey, the link between her spirituality, and the love she felt in her relationship with the divine, were the things that made the difference.

Near the end of the interview I asked Jaya what she would want to tell her daughter, if she ever has one, about her own relationship to her body. She paused for a while, sifting thoughts and ideas, and pulling them out of her mind like a magician pulling a multicolored scarf from the sleeve. "I love to feel and know that I am healthy," she said. Then she pulled some more: "I don't depend on [men] to tell me that I'm valuable." Then, as she circled back to our conversation about God and faith, she said, "This [culture] will never completely accept me, there will always be something wrong with me, so why would I go [into a battle I know I will fail]? That is just a battle I will lose if I try to compare myself, but I know that I am guaranteed [success, safety, security, acceptance, and victory] with God."

BEING SEEN AND BEING LOVED

I had probably been coming to see her for several weeks at this point when Liz said something that made me feel pride in myself for the first time in a striking amount of time. She said, *women with eating disorders are philosopher queens*. I still don't really know what she meant when she said this, if she made it up, or what she hoped it would help me know. But what I remember feeling when she said that is that someone saw all of the horrible parts of the disorder, and still had something good to say. Maybe *philosopher queen* is a putdown to someone else; maybe it means someone who overthinks things. But to me, the words themselves, and the way she spoke them in that moment, it was like she saw me as a prophet, a mystic, a poet, a royal. It made me think that maybe the reason I was sick wasn't because I was weak, shallow, self-absorbed, or not loved enough by my mother. I for the first time considered in that moment that one of the things that was my greatest gift was also part of what made me suffer: I feel and think deeply. I am sensitive, to what is shown to me, hidden from me, to what others feel, and what is all around. And from very young I have too often felt and pondered the immense pain and fear of utter aloneness in this world. I have long since thought about all the ways that Liz's words are true, and not true. It seems to be a string of words that I've worn like a necklace for over a decade—looking at myself in the mirror and noticing this thing, dangling there that wasn't before, sometimes complimenting my features, other times an afterthought.
Maybe I am a philosopher queen, maybe not. But I am so much more than my weight, than my breast size, than if I fit into the jeans I wore before I started my doctoral program, or what men walking by me on the street think of me. And as Liz taught me, I am also more than my pain or the things that I do battle with. Liz is not God, but she showed me

more about how God sees me, and that has been an important part of my healing. I believe that I am loved, valuable, and worthy, and that it is not a mistake that I take up space in this world.

REFLECTION QUESTIONS

- What would it mean to know I was ultimately loved, and did not have to earn that from someone, nor could someone else take it away?
- What are my faith and spiritual practices, and how can I draw from those as a source of compassion and affection for myself and my body?
- When have I felt most alive? What are the most meaningful parts of life?
- What are the things I love about myself?
- Who are the strong women in my life who I can turn to when I need to know that I am loved, and not alone?
- What are my thoughts about the "something more" piece discussed in this chapter? How does it fit with me, or not?

▶ If you have a daughter...
  - What are ways I can notice and celebrate my individuality and uniqueness?
  - What are the things I love about my daughter? What do I want to tell my daughter about the "something more" in life?
  - Underneath all of the things that she does that I disagree with are things that make my daughter unique, and lovable: what are those things, and how can I find more ways to celebrate those things with her?
  - What can I teach my daughter about surrounding her with people who love her well?

NINE

WHEN IT'S MESSY: THE IMPORTANCE OF FEELING

"There is a crack in everything, that's how the light gets in."

–LEONARD COHEN

This is a chapter about pain: pain within us, pain among us and around us, and the healing, feeling, and dealings of it. On the day I had written in my calendar that I would start to write this chapter I slept in, did my laundry, bought groceries, moved my eyes down several pages of a book that I didn't actually read, and then sat at my computer. Nothing happened. It's probably more accurate to say that I didn't let anything happen. I felt agitated, anxious, like a subtle electric current running through my body. I couldn't sit, I couldn't write—not like this. So I got up again, finding dishes to wash and then a very important and distracting article to read. This was the day I would write what you were meant to be reading now, red marker circling the box representing this day.

"You're avoiding this," said the one part of my mind that was not avoiding.

I had written the rest of the book months ago. It seemed that after completing the research, defending the thesis, publishing the formal manuscript in a respected research journal, writing again the stories of other women I had let steep both my dreams and waking thoughts for years, that writing would be effortless. And for the most part the other chapters of the book flowed freely. It was like my thoughts, as they were happening, were suddenly transported through my fingertips and onto the page. But then this chapter came, and things stopped. I had come up with a story, or a few, to make sense of the energetic change: "I'm a student, I should work on homework," "the book can wait, I'll do that when I have more time," and "I'm working too much and I need to rest—I'm a therapist, you know, and would want my clients to know that I take care of myself in all the ways I remind them to." But when I would make time to write, this chapter in particular, that familiar electricity feeling would come back—either slowly creeping up, or hitting me all at once, sending waves of "stop, do something else" and "go watch a movie" through my thoughts. Now it was the day when I had purposefully gotten rid of all of the things that normally added to the story that I couldn't write this chapter now. But I found that every time I sat down to write, I was suddenly preoccupied with an assortment of tasks which would subtly distract me until I came up with something else to distract me further. But in a moment of painful realization, the quiet thought broke through, "You're avoiding this."

So I did what I would tell anyone else to do: I got quiet on the inside and the outside. I put the things in my hands down, and I lay down onto the floor on my back with my arms open wide on my sides, and had a meeting. With myself. Usually this involves putting on some sort of comfortable elastic waistband pants, hair in a ponytail, and all the lights off. Although I wasn't quite sure what was going on, I wasn't going to keep running from it. If parts of my mind had actual voices, here is what that meeting would have sounded like:

You're avoiding this.

No, I don't really think so, there are just so many other things that need to be done

Oh really? How come you feel that anxious electricity feeling whenever you think about this chapter? And how come that feeling goes away whenever you do something else?

... I think you're right, but I'm not sure what I'm avoiding.

Well, let's talk about it, we'll figure it out together. Tell me what the chapter is about?

Pain. Feeling pain, dealing with pain, all of it.

... Oh, I see (laughs, playfully). And you're wondering what you are avoiding? It sounds like it would be really hard to write that chapter, given, you know, how you almost killed yourself trying to get rid of it, or run from it, for so many years. It makes a lot of sense to me that sitting down to really feel it would be scary.

(Silence) I'm afraid.

Afraid of what?

I'm afraid that I won't have anything to say, that I am a fraud. I see it now; I'm doing what I always did when I was sick. I ran. I stayed busy. I lied to myself and to other people. I made up excuses. I lived in the fear of what would happen when I couldn't run anymore from the things that hurt most. And now I'm doing it again. How can I have anything meaningful to write about pain, and the feeling of it, when I obviously don't know how to do that? I'm afraid that when people read this, they will see that I don't really know what I'm talking about—that my heart is still so messy, and that even though I'm "recovered", sometimes I feel like I'm a "mess" and need to grieve when an old pair of pants won't zip up. When I think about it, I'm also afraid that people will read this and will think that I'm perfect, or have it all figured out, and I'll have something I'm responsible for creating in their minds that I can't live up to. I don't want that either. I don't know what I want, or what I'm trying to say. But writing about pain makes me feel my own. And for some reason, the hurting, and what I've done in the past, and what I do now, to run from the hurting, makes it so much harder to believe that I could offer something to others that might help them do it. (Cue floods of tears.)

(Silence). I am with you. I'm not going anywhere. I will lay here with you until you don't need to lay here anymore. (Pause) Thank you for telling me all of that. I am proud of you. It hurts to feel our pain. It also hurts to keep running from it, mostly because we can't really do that. I am so proud of you for being honest, for laying down with me, and telling me what you were scared of. It's hard to face things that are scary—you're doing it. So you put it off for a while, maybe that is what you needed to be ready. And when you were ready, you heard my voice reminding you that you were in fact running from something.

Don't you think that makes me a hypocrite?

No (laughs), it makes you human.

So what now?

Let's go write.

172

About what? I haven't even thought about that.

This. Write about what's happening right now. Tell the truth.

What do you think people would think about me?

What is that thing you always say, those words you sing with your heart over and over again in therapy? Rumi's words …

"Tear off the mask, your face is glorious." … (Put one hand on my stomach, one hand on my chest—and gently press, feeling a few breaths cycle in and out.) Ok. Let's go write.

The irony wasn't lost on me. I had wanted to sit down and write about pain, about feeling it, and what to do when it hits us over the head or sneaks up on us, and how that all has to do with our bodies, our relationships with other people—all of it. But I got stuck, overwhelmed by writing about something that evidently is still hard for me. In having a meeting with myself I remembered so many of the things it took me forever to learn—I can do this, I am not alone, I can tell the truth about how I feel, I don't need to be perfect to be valuable, and that the most authentic version of me is the most beautiful one. It was remembering all those things that helped me endure the discomfort of sitting with this pain, while writing what you are reading now.

WHY IT'S HARD TO FEEL

The women I interviewed didn't talk much about their experiences of feeling pain. They shared moments of shame about their appearance and their bodies, acne, cellulite, not getting their periods when everyone else had them, or being slow to develop and feeling like a child while everyone else was becoming a woman. Some of the mothers described crippling anxiety, or experiencing abuse at the hands of a parent, or partner. But overall there wasn't much in great detail in the interviews about how they got through the messy pain. It wasn't something I realized until now that I would want to ask them. It doesn't mean that they never felt pain, or didn't have important things to say about feeling it, and moving through it, I just didn't think to ask. When crafting the questions that I was going to ask, I did not know just how important emotions and feeling them are in helping us love ourselves, our bodies.

The more I read about our experiences of and in our bodies as women, the more therapy I do with other people, and of my own, the more evident the link becomes. Pain is not fun to feel. That is true when we know how to actually let ourselves feel it. But what is becoming even more clear through research in the field of interpersonal neurobiology, affective neuroscience, and attachment work is that some of us don't actually know how to feel hard things.[46] Some of us were never taught. When the social-emotional parts of our brain were being shaped during our early years, and we arrived in a foreign land of sadness, anger, shame, fear, loneliness (insert any other challenging emotion here), we weren't lovingly shown the path back to a state of restfulness, calm, and ease.[47] So later in life, when the heavy, painful, messy stuff comes up, the experience is literally so overwhelming that the only thing to do is shove it down, push it away, numb it, cut ourselves, or run as fast as possible to the fridge or the liquor.

Remember that all of this is happening in a culture where we're told as women (and men!) that emotions are bad, they are unreasonable, a sign of weakness, and decidedly unlogical (mostly because they've historically been seen as confirming the hysterical nature of women). We're told and shown repeatedly that showing our painful emotions make others uncomfortable—"so keep your pain private," if you can feel it at all. Stack that on top of a world which tells us that controlling our bodies, shrinking, shaping, disappearing, more of this part, less of that part, is what will make it "all good"– it is kind of miraculous that all of us do not have eating disorders when I look at it that way.

EMOTIONS IN THE BODY

As I wrote in several of the other chapters, having a dualistic split of the mind and the body impairs our full experience of ourselves as humans, and leads us treating ourselves and others as objects which we carry around our minds. This can make it seem like our minds are being good by trying to control what we do with our bodies, which are bad. But when we split ourselves in two like this, it further impairs our ability to feel. Or, more accurately, erases the way we think about the goodness of our bodies, how our bodies invite us into a fuller and more rich experience of life. It took me a long time to learn that, contrary to what I'd always thought, our emotions exist in our bodies, the primary more universal ones anyway. But in order to really grasp this it's helpful to know that our brains and our bodies are not distinct and independently functioning aspects of the self. Together our brain and body are interdependent in their ability to function, working together at every moment to help us be the person we are, to think, feel, react, and exist the way we do. Some researchers, theorists, and clinicians, especially those who work in the field of trauma, actually use the word brain/body to come up with a term that adequately captures the complexity of who we are as people, and what it's like for us to move through the world and experience life. What we learn from research in the fields of affective neuroscience and somatic psychology is that when we feel a certain emotion, our body is wired to respond accordingly—that allows us to respond appropriately, especially in situations when we feel threatened.[48] If we saw a bear coming towards us while we were hiking in the woods, we would feel fear. The fear immediately has an effect on our nervous system, increasing oxygen to our muscles and increasing our heart rates so we can get ourselves out of the threatening situation. It happens automatically. What is really interesting is that although there is some variability, people generally experience emotions through their bodies in the same patterns—with feelings like emotion, disgust, anger, pride, and fear creating generally the same physiological experiences of activation and deactivation, such as

175

heat in the chest, or tingling throughout the body. Neuroscientist Antonio Damasio has been talking about this for a long time in his work, and even goes so far as to say that each emotion has a physiological signature, and it's our mind's awareness of that specific pattern, or signature, that helps us know what we're feeling.[49] And knowing what we're feeling is an important part of being able to deal with it—to emotionally regulate. But if we're dissociated from our body, if we believe it's bad, if we don't even believe we need to listen to it, it makes it harder to take the information we learn through our body and use it to help us be healthiest, and most fully alive.

TOO MUCH FEELING AND NOT ENOUGH FEELING

Depending on what it's like to be us, and what we've been through in our lives, we can vary in how much and what kind of emotions dominate our experience. Often these are shaped by our early experiences, how we were responded to and interacted with, right from the beginning, with the people in our lives, family, friends, teachers, etc. It's normal for people who had experiences growing up of danger and unsafety, especially when this was reoccurring or consistent, to feel a lot of anxiety later in life for seemingly no reason. Or, if we learned[50] (even if not intended) that we were only good for the things we did, our accomplishments, appearance, or whatever, or that we weren't loveable just as we are, we might experience shame. These are just some broad stroke examples of how our early environments (or traumatic events later in life) shape our feelings about ourselves, and what it means to be us in the world. And based on that, some people end up experiencing really loud and painful emotions on a more regular basis than others. It's also really normal for our emotions to get so big, or for us to have learned that they are so unsafe and so unwelcome, that it's like we shut off from them altogether. The consequence of this is that we move through life part-alive, part-present, part-us. There are fancy words for this, and it depends on the researcher or clinician to decide what's most suitable in those situations. I like to use the words dissociation, numbing, or detachment, to talk about when this happens in myself and other people. What we do know in research is that people who spend a lot of time in "the feelings are too big" place or the "I don't feel at all" place have difficulty with a lot of things, and tend to do things to try and not feel so much, or nothing at all.

What researchers have shown repeatedly[51] is that people who have difficulty with emotional regulation, or don't know how to respond to, feel, and manage their emotions in healthy ways, often experience depression, anxiety, unhealthy eating behaviors and eating disorders, self-harm, and substance use. It is too painful to live in the "feeling too much" land, and it can feel like we're not even alive when we live in the "I can't feel anything" land. The sad things about this, is that for many of us who have cut off feelings to try to numb our pain, we ended up cutting of more than just the pain, and we lost the good feelings too. In her work, Brené Brown has clearly articulated that we cannot numb selectively. In an effort to numb the bad, we also end up numbing the good. When we are afraid of feeling, we don't just limit the depth of the pain we feel, but also the heights of joy.

EMOTIONAL REGULATION

In the academic and clinical communities, the word we used to describe the process of learning to come back to restfulness and ease when we've been in the "feeling too much" land, or the "I don't feel anything at all" land, is called *emotional regulation*. It is our learned ability to notice and experience our emotions, and then respond to them accordingly. It is like an internal thermostat, which notices and then makes changes accordingly, to help us stay emotionally within a range of feelings that is tolerable, productive, and socially appropriate (that range is called the window of tolerance—a term coined by Dan Siegel). Usually this involves some degree of skill—which fortunately we can learn over time—and helps us respond both spontaneously and in delaying spontaneous responses and experiences when appropriate. Most of us use at least some emotional regulation strategies throughout the day, like taking a deep breath when we are getting overwhelmed, or rubbing our neck after a stressful meeting to help ourselves let go of the tension. For example, if Jessica is on the way to a big event that is making her feel anxious, because she is anxious she is running late for the bus and getting more and more anxious and overwhelmed. Her ability to practice emotional regulation in that moment might start with her noticing her anxiety because of her racing heart, shortness of breath, and scattered thoughts. Having noticed this, she might stop, call a taxi instead of rushing for the bus (and getting even more anxious if she misses it), and take a few moments to breathe and talk herself down with a kind and encouraging inner dialogue.

The reason that some of us reach for food when we are feeling overwhelmed, lonely, or sad is that food, especially food high in sugars, releases serotonin—a powerful neurotransmitter (brain chemical) that can lift our mood temporarily and affect lots of other parts of our brain. And our brain forms associations really quickly—learning that doing that certain action made me feel better, for a little while. So the next time we are feeling overwhelmed, lonely, or sad, we're more likely to do the thing that worked last time. Then that becomes the thing we do: eating to feel better. But we can eat so much that it starts us make to feel out of control or gain weight. If we are afraid of gaining weight (since we have learned from young that being anything other than thin is not ok at all), it might feel like the only way we can stop of the out of control feeling, or the weight gain, to exercise compulsively, purge, or eat even more. This might, for the moment feel like it helps with shame, or makes us seem more in control. And as so many authors on the topic of binge eating write, unlike people, food does not talk back, it will never emotionally abandon you, and it never asks for anything in return.

Although it depends on the person, our most current understanding of eating disorders is that they are highly linked to a limited ability to emotionally regulate. Prominent emotional patterns are thought to show up in the people who struggle with each kind of eating disorder, anorexia, bulimia, and binge eating. But generally it appears as though most people who struggle with disordered eating have challenges noticing, responding to, and managing emotions.[52] But this, as I wrote about in the earlier chapters, it is inadequate to consider these emotional regulation issues without also examining the sociopolitical context within which they exist. The culture rewards women for disappearing, or conforming, to the beauty ideals. Women who don't meet beauty ideals are either invisible or shamed, sometimes in society, but almost always within themselves, adding onto the tide of emotions, which may feel overwhelming, trapping her within a seemingly endless cycle.

LEARNING EMOTIONAL REGULATION

It is hopeful, empowering, and redemptive to know that we can learn to emotionally regulate. It's not too late to do this for yourself, or if you're a parent, it's not too late to start thinking about doing these things with your children.

- Before you do anything else, try thinking of yourself as a whole person where brain and body are actually connected. Try and notice how immediate it is for you to think about wiggling your toes, and actually doing it. Try imagining that your fingers are connected to your brain. If you pinch the skin on your hand, notice that it hurts. Try being thankful in that moment that pain is something your brain and body do together to try to keep you safe.

- Start paying attention to which specific emotions you feel, and when you're feeling them. Notice the difference (in body, thought, action) between anxiety and excitement, or sadness and loneliness, or shame and guilt. Notice if there are emotions which are really hard to identify when you experience them, but are easy to understand intellectually. If you aren't sure, you could start with broader categories and ask yourself questions: do I feel "up" or "low," is the "up" or "down" enjoyable or not?

- When you notice a specific emotion, see if you can think of the emotion like a geologist looks at a rock: be curious, try and see it from all angles, but be careful not to judge it.
- Think about growing up, and what emotions would best characterize your experience. What emotions did you see most from your parents, or family members? Which ones did you see least? Which ones did they help you with and did they invite you to share with them? Which ones were not allowed, or were supposed to happen in isolation? What were you told or shown to do when you were sad? Or afraid?
- Start paying attention to specific emotions in other people. When you're at work, on transit, in class, or at the lineup in the grocery store, see if you can notice how people are feeling by how assessing their body language, tone of voice if they're speaking, and facial expressions. In your head (not out loud) see if you can figure out what combinations of emotions someone might be feeling, like scared and embarrassed, or excited and nervous.
- Notice when things feel uncomfortable, and accept it. It is normal to be in awkward situations; we have all said "no" to someone trying to sell us something, and they keep persisting. Or at a dinner party when there is a lull in the conversation. Notice the awkwardness in your body, and what specifically is happening that feels uncomfortable. This is not about when someone is sexually assaulting you, or you are unsafe and being violated in any way. But in the minor situations which occur on a regular basis which are actually part of being human, see if you can notice the discomfort, and actually step into it, seeking to understand it and explore the experience of it in your body, and the thoughts that come along, being curious instead of judgmental. Notice

how much you avoid these situations, and if you could try and lean into them instead. This is called *mindfulness*, and there are a lot of resources out there to help you learn if you want to.

- Notice anxiety, and be friendly towards it, without letting it control you all the time. As in the story above about the meeting I had with myself, notice what you feel, and see if you can explore where it comes from, and then try and do it anyway. Don't go so far that you create panic, but challenge yourself a little bit to prove to the anxiety that it doesn't have all the power. When we don't do things that make us anxious, it feels good right away, but over time it can increase our anxiety, and make us anxious about more things than the thing that originally made us anxious. For example, when going to a party makes you feel anxious, notice that feeling, and see if you can make it there and just walk through the door. Then if you need to, step outside, and see if you can let the anxiety settle a bit. If you feel better, go back inside, if not, go home. Next time a party comes up, remind yourself that you can go, and try and stay five minutes before you leave.

- Learn how to meditate. If you haven't done this before, try starting with the breathing exercise described below and just notice your breathing for a minute or so. When you notice you're distracted, bring your attention back to your breathing, noticing the feelings in your body when you fill and empty your lungs. Try doing this every day for a few days, then expand the time to five minutes. Don't expect to be perfect at it; for a lot of people this is more like a brain workout than a relaxation exercise. It can be helpful to think about something in particular, or focus on your breathing, or listen to music, or an audio track which guides your thoughts. See if over time you can get distracted less, or bring yourself back to your focal point more quickly. Try to picture yourself in an imaginary peaceful place, outside of time, and where you are sure that you will be safe.

- Get enough sleep, and make sure to exercise a healthy amount. Both of these are known to help support the parts of our mind that we need to be able to access our emotional regulation skills when we need them, or stop big feelings from feeling so big in the first place. A mix of cardiovascular exercise, yoga, and stretching seems to be helpful.

Some of the activities listed below are particularly helpful for teaching children and teenagers of most ages. So try them yourself, and if you have kids of any age, try showing them how to do these things too. I like to keep a list of things that work for me when I'm overwhelmed (right now I keep it digitally so I can access it from anywhere). That way, if you don't have this book with you, you can just pull out the list.

When big, painful, and overwhelming feelings come up:

- Try taking several deep breaths. Make sure that the breath out is longer than the breath in. Try breathing in for six seconds, and out for ten seconds, pausing when your lungs are full of air, and again when they are totally empty. See if you can breathe right into the pit of your stomach, like your gut is a balloon filling with air.
- Try going to the peaceful place you go to in your mind when you meditate. Say a prayer, think of a special and relaxing memory, or picture a relaxing image.
- Try giving yourself a hug, or shoulder rub. The trick here is to think of this in two parts, then add them together. First, while hugging yourself, imagine being the person getting a hug, feel yourself wrapped up in someone's arms, warm, and cared for. Then switch to imagining being the person

giving the hug, your arms wrapping around someone who is needing to feel cared for right now. Then, do them both— try and hold yourself in the place mentally where you are aware of both giving and receiving the touch.

- Tell yourself something kind but true. This works best when we do this in a calm and encouraging tone either inside our heads, or out loud. Some of the examples I like to use: I can handle this. I have been through many difficult situations before, and I can get through this too. What do I need to do to take care of myself right now? What does the wise woman have to say? I will take a minute to feel this, I know it will not kill me. I can ask for help if I need it. I am valuable, no matter what. I am enough, just as I am. I don't need to be perfect to be lovable. How can I honor myself most in this situation right now? This feeling of intensity can only last so long, so if nothing else, I can wait it out.

- If there is someone around who loves you, who you feel safe with, ask them to talk, give a hug, tell you a funny story, tell you any story at all, or to look you in the eye and tell you what they love about you. If they are not with you, just think about them and what they might say to you.

- Try counting backwards from a very big number by seven or thirteen until you notice that your body and thoughts have settled a bit.

- Go for a walk, or run. Stretch or do yoga. Move yourself— dance, or flap your hands, something to get the intensity out if you need to.

- Try writing your feelings in a journal. Some people like writing in their journal about what feels hard as a way of getting it "out"; other people like to write a letter to themselves as a way of talking themselves "down." One thing I've found helpful is to imagine having two parts of you write back and forth to each other. Kind of like the "self-meeting" I wrote about at the beginning of the chapter. Let one part of you talk about the messy stuff, and have the other part provide comfort. (This can be a really productive and insightful exercise to try with yourself on days when loving yourself, your body, seems particularly challenging).

- Do something kind for yourself: make tea, have a bath, draw or make art, do something that feels soothing and nurturing.
- Connect with nature: walk barefoot or lie on the grass, hug a tree, watch birds, or run your hand through a stream.

Learning to emotionally regulate is an incredible gift you can give yourself, and can help us prevent eating disorders and enjoy the experience of being ourselves in our bodies more. It helps us feel the hard things, but also helps us reconnect to the good things. When we numb feelings, we numb them all, so when we get them back, we get back the good ones too. Because feelings are in our body, feeling good things can help us connect with our bodies in an enjoyable and positive way. It is something I want for all of us as women. If you are a mother, you have the added job of helping your kids learn how to do it. It's hard to help other people learn to do things we don't know how to do, so taking this work seriously for yourself is an incredible gesture of love for those you are raising, and those around you. If you are really struggling with this, learning how to do it in a relationship is a really good idea. Try finding a therapist who knows how to do this work, and other body-based or emotion-focused work too.

All of that stuff you're reading about, mothers, daughters, emotions, our inner relationship with ourselves, helping raise daughters who love their bodies—it all takes place in a world which tells us to look, act, speak a certain way as girls and women. I wish I completely understood the specific connection between pain and eating disorders and body hatred, so that I could show it to you under a microscope, or that you could hold it in your hands and feel how real it is. But as for right now all I can say is that the links are there, although at times fuzzy in terms of how they first showed up in my own life. Maybe I was feeling overwhelming shame that made me want to disappear long before I directed that shame towards my body. Maybe managing my body, depriving it, abusing it, might have been a socially acceptable way to find some control, or something that felt like I could do to make things not hurt so bad inside. But if we *are* our bodies, and we are hurting, overwhelmed, anxious, afraid, and feel shame about who we are, I believe that that will translate to all of us, to how we think about, behave, talk, and care for all parts of us.

UP FROM THE BOTTOM

I think that what got me sick so long ago is that when I felt pain—mine, someone else's, any at all, really—it was like I had tied a boulder to my ankles and thrown it overboard, into an ocean that had no bottom. Even the idea of hitting the bottom of the ocean seemed to be a relief, because then it would be over, instead of the sting of not knowing while falling further and further away from what I knew. I can only speculate as to why I felt so much pain. Long before Liz called me one of the "philosopher queens," I thought a lot about death, life, what makes us matter, what makes us lovable, and felt the feelings of those thoughts very deeply.

I know that my mom did her very best to help me with those big feelings, but I think that some of them were so big for me that they were too big for her. Because I am her baby, she saw and felt the pain I was feeling, and it overwhelmed her too. As an adult I've gotten to know more and more about what it was like for my mom growing up in her family. The short way to say this is that growing up, she was almost never safe, never shown how valuable she was, never allowed to feel—certainly not feelings that were uncomfortable or demanded something from others. And years later, she has two children, and I understand now that the best she could have ever given to me was to break the patterns of pain and hurt in the way that she was treated, and to do her best to love me differently. She did an absolutely incredible job of turning the ashes of her own upbringing into the beauty of how she parented me. In putting energy into giving me the ladder to a different life than she had, there were some things that she didn't know how to do, or that she didn't get to do as well as she would have liked. When my feelings were big, and scary, and messy, it was like the boulder tied to my ankle got looped around hers too. And sometimes the other way around. Either way, we sometimes got stuck in this emotional drowning experience, and she didn't help me untie the rope from my ankle. She didn't know how. No one ever taught her. I know that her mother, my grandmother, did not know how, because I learned that no one ever taught her. The cycle goes on and on and on, until someone is courageous, and supported, and privileged enough to be able to make a change. My mother broke the patterns of her in her family because she is tough as nails, and has done her work, and has a heart made of the most precious gems. And she loved me enough, even when she didn't give me what I needed to feel and heal and work with my emotions, so that I could go on to one day give my children the experience of someone showing them how to untie the knot from around their ankles. My mom loved me well enough that I can do better than she did. Even though I struggled with an eating disorder, my mom gave me the ladder she never had, and I want to do the same for my children one day.

MAYNE ISLAND

A little while after I started writing this chapter, having gently but persistently escorted myself through the discomfort of encountering my avoidance, I went away for a few days on a writing retreat. I have found it's easier to connect with myself, and then write from that place of connectedness, when there aren't as many distractions around. I was on a little island not too far from my home, tucked under some blankets on a chair pulled up next to a blazing fire in a little cabin I'd rented for the weekend. All alone, only the noise of the cracking burning wood, I was sitting, thinking about all of this, reading and rereading what I'd written, and I suddenly noticed a pressure building under my sternum. I observed it climb higher, sweep out into my chest, then bubble into my throat. At first it felt like I was choking and I felt myself nervously resisting the aliveness of the sensation. As soon as I gave in, it shot out my eyes in drops of water. Out of nowhere, so it seemed, I was weeping. Out of my eyes, coursing through my body, were all sorts of feelings. I felt like I was feeling sadness and joy and pride for my mother—for all the pain she has been through and how courageous she has been. I was feeling grief for our relationship, and how much it must have hurt her to see me hurt, and how much I wished she would have known what to do, and known what I needed, even though I didn't. I felt guilt that one of the only ways I knew how to get healthy, to figure out who I was on my own, was to push her away. I felt fear that when she would read this book that she would think I don't love her as much as I do. I felt the swells of gratitude that healing was happening in my life. I felt the pain, and fullness, and richness, of being alive. All at once, all messy, all of the feelings. They were all there. It was like I got so far into the feeling of things that I hit a fork in the feeling road; I had cried enough to take the edge off, to really let myself know I was not running from anything. I remember looking around, kind of getting my bearings, almost to see if someone had snuck up to the window and was watching me sob. Then I realized again the irony, that I was writing a chapter about letting myself feel, and doing that in a healthy way, and not numbing anymore. I made a choice in that moment that felt like coming up for a big breath of air, before going back under to feel again. And this time I really let it happen. I remember opening my arms up and throwing my head back, and letting my whole body shake as I cried. It felt like a profound moment of healing, or realization, to know I could trust myself to feel that deeply without fearing getting lost in it, without fearing it at all. I probably cried for over half an hour, although time seemed to mean nothing when I was finally with myself without shame. And it felt good too, like a valve I had closed at age twelve was opened. My young self with so much shame and insecurity and pain, who didn't have my mother to help her find her way back to the surface, had me now, and I could help her feel the pain, and come through it. When whatever that was that happened was done happening, some spiritual or emotional cleansing of sorts, I sent a message to my mom. It said, "I can't remember what I told you, but I'm away this weekend on Mayne Island to finish my book. I'm thinking about you a lot, and thankful for how you've loved me, even when it hurt you, even when it hurt me. I want you to read the book before it goes to press so we can talk about what needs to be talked about, if anything, and so you feel safe with what I'm writing. I found this poem and burst into tears reading it:

"Like flowers ache for spring
my heart craves my mother
more than anything."

–Rupi Kaur

I have so much ambivalence in our relationships, and desperately want to be close to you, but feel sometimes like I don't know how to do that without being who I think you want me to be, or who you are, or pushing away from you and just being me. So I'm sorry. But I love you. and I never want to miss a chance to tell you that."

Shortly after she wrote back, "My dear daughter Hillary, I love you, and know that you love me. I can see it in your eyes, and feel it in your hugs. I hope that someday you will be able to feel and to know how much I love you. I look forward to reading your book, because it's you: your writing, your thoughts, your ideas. I am proud of who you are. Be proud of yourself. I love you." This was not the first of this kind of conversation between us. We were healing, together. No more avoiding. No more numbing, no more of me expecting for her to heal me anymore; that was no longer her job, it's now mine.

To all of you reading this, whatever you did get might have been the best your mother could have given you at that time. Maybe, just maybe, she was doing better than was done for her. And it's probable that you didn't get what you needed either. That can all be true all at the same time.

And now you have a choice, about doing something with what you have been given, and making it your job to keep the work going. Even if your mother hated her body, you don't have to. And even if you hate yours (you don't have to always), your daughter doesn't have to. One of the best ways we can love ourselves is to give ourselves what we didn't have. And one of the best ways we can love our children, and those close to us, is to give ourselves, and each other, what we didn't have. We don't need to be perfect to do any of this. We can do it all, as we are.

EPILOGUE: A LETTER TO MY DAUGHTER

Dear Daughter, I don't know how old you or I will be when you are reading this, but I am so glad that you are. Even though while I'm writing this I don't know who you are while you are reading this, I know that I love you. Even now, while you are still a dream to me. I have so many things to say, things that I want you to always know, things that I want us all to know:

- You do not have to be anyone else's version of you to be lovable, and worthy of belonging. That includes me, and my ideas for you. I love psychology and helping other people heal, but if what makes you feel alive is blowing glass, or working as a welder, writing plays, or computer programming, I want you to know that the world is better off when you are the fullest and most alive version of you, not anyone else's version of you.

- As long as you are not hurting yourself, or other people, I hope that you have the courage to try things that scare you, things that make you feel alive, creative, and connected to yourself and other people.

- I hope that I can show you that mistakes are part of learning, and that you do not have to be perfect to be valuable and know that you belong. Making mistakes is a part of trying things, and trying things is such an important part of growth, discovery, and adventure.

- I am sorry. I hope I say this a lot. I want to show you that it's ok to say it a lot, that part of being a healthy human means recognizing and taking responsibility for our mistakes. I want it to be easy for you to say sorry when you grow up, so that you can say sorry to the people you love, and help them heal. I am sorry for the ways I have hurt you. I am sorry for the ways I didn't know how to make it better when you were hurting. I am sorry for letting my hang-ups and fears get in the way of your freedom and creativity. I am sorry for when I made you think that my frustration and confusion was because you weren't good enough. And I am sorry for not saying "I am sorry" enough.

- You don't ever need to shrink down in body, voice, thought, or action to be lovable. You already are lovable. It is ok to feel guilty if something you do hurts yourself, someone else, or the earth, but you never have to feel shame for being who you are.

- It is ok to feel lots of big emotions, and even lots of big emotions at the same time. You can come to me to talk about them, and figure out what to do about them, and we will learn together how to move through the difficult things in life together. You never have to feel bad about asking for help, and you never have to feel bad about sharing the scary things with the people who love you and are safe for you. Being vulnerable, especially with the right person or people, can be one of the most important paths to healing.

- There are stories about being a woman that your culture will tell you, and you have a choice about what you do with those stories. You don't have to take them in blindly. Think hard about those stories, and if they help you feel big and wild and free, or small, shamed, and scared. And if those stories don't fit with what you've learned about what it means to be alive in a good and beautiful way in the world, then you can write your own story about being a woman, or find other people to help you write a new story. You may feel like you

191

don't fit in, or belong, especially when you are thinking for yourself. But I promise, you dear one, you are never alone—it may just take time to find the proof.

- Your body does not make you valuable. And at the same time, your body is an important part of who you are—it is what makes you alive, capable, and strong in the world, able to get, give, and make love, and hold the ones you love. You are a human with a divine spark that lives inside of you always, and you are not an object which anyone is allowed to use.

- I have no idea what you look like, but I know that you are beautiful. I know that because beauty comes in so many different ways. I know that when you are most fully yourself, no matter what that means, there will be something about you that draws people towards you.

- If you can help it, try not to compare yourself with other people around you, especially when it comes to your looks. Let them be them, and you be you. If you do notice the differences and similarities between you and other people, be curious and full of wonder—taking joy in the special things they offer the world without worrying that takes away from the special things you offer to the world.

- You are not a mistake.

- You are totally and completely enough, just as you are.

ACKNOWLEDGMENTS

It is only because of the brave women who share their stories with me that this book exists. Thank you for reaching out, telling the truth, and letting me into your lives. In the words of Clarissa Pinkola Estés, "One of the most calming and powerful actions you can do to intervene in a stormy world is to stand up and show your soul." To my master's thesis supervisor, mentor, and friend, Janelle Kwee, you have been my hero in so many ways—a midwife for the research and this book from the beginning, guiding, cheering, and loving it all into being. Thank you for letting my mind and heart flourish through the safety and guidance of your mentorship. You have been, and always will be, a precious gift to me. To Ramani, without whom this book would still be waiting to be written— your enthusiasm and investment in me and in this book was the spark I needed. Thank you for all of the time and love you have poured into helping this book exist. To me, you are proof that there are good, loving, passionate, and wise people in the world with mind-blowing generosity. To Kelsey, you were the first person I told about the book, and the first person to read it all the way through—your presence on this journey with me has been invaluable, and your friendship through it has kept my heart safe, soft, and open. To everyone who has helped me through Post Hill Press, Anthony, Billie, and the rest of the team, I could not have done this without you.

This book has been loved into being by my community. All of my successes are the fruit of your love and wisdom. You know who you are. Thank you for being with me through my pain and holding my hand and walking with me towards healing and growth. To the women in my life who have been with me through the fire: Alexandra, Sarah, Jess, Melissa,

Catherine, and Krista. To Alastair [insert hilarious/witty/sarcastic comment here], thank you for your expertise, and benevolent direction. To Dad, thanks for being so many things for this book all wrapped into one: editor, advisor, hugger, cheerleader. Thank you for your thoughtfulness; it has been precious for me to have you with me in this all. Nano—it's pretty cool to have my childhood hero also be my big brother. I love you. Kevin, my heart. You have been through it all, and fiercely you have loved me—teaching me how to love myself and waking up something sacred that we now hold between us. All of my success are ours, my love.

To my mother, whose body was once my home, and whose love is like a melody in my soul:

"I will say it is so: The first voice I heard belonged to my mother. It was her voice I listened to from the womb; from the moment my head emerged into this world; from the moment I was pushed out, then placed on her belly before the umbilicus was cut; from the moment when she cradled me in her arms. My mother spoke to me: 'Hello, little one. You are here, I am here.' I will say it is so: My mother's voice is a lullaby in my cells. When I am still, my body feels her breathing."

–Terry Tempest Williams, *When Women Were Birds*

ENDNOTES

1   Corning, A. F., Gondoli, D. M., Bucchianeri, M. M., & Salafia, E. H. B. "Preventing the development of body issues in adolescent girls through intervention with their mothers." *Body Image*, 7(4) (2010): 289-295.

2   Haines, J., Neumark-Sztainer, D., Perry, C. L., Hannan, P. J., & Levine, M. P. "V. I. K. (very important kids): A school-based program designed to reduce teasing and unhealthy weight-control behaviors." *Health Education Research*, 21 (2006): 884–895.

3   Smolak, L., Levine, M., & Schermer, F. "Parental input and weight concerns among elementary school children." *International Journal of Eating Disorders*, 25 (1999): 339–343.

4   Hardit, S. & Hannum, J. "Attachment, the tripartite influence model, and the development of body dissatisfaction." *Body Image*, 9 (2012): 469-475.

5   Cash, T. F., Theriault, J., & Annis, N. W. "Body image in an interpersonal con-text: Adult attachment, fear of intimacy, and social anxiety." *Journal of Social and Clinical Psychology*, 23 (2004): 89–103.

    Cheng, H. L., & Malinkcrodt, B. "Parental bonds, anxious attachment, media internalization, and body image dissatisfaction:

Exploring a mediation model." *Journal of Counseling Psychology, 56* (2009): 365–375.

Greenwood, D., & Pietromonaco, P. R. "The interplay among attachment orientation, idealized media images of women, and body dissatisfaction: A social psychological analysis." In L. Shrum (Ed.), *The Psychology of Entertainment Media: Blurring the Lines Between Entertainment and Persuasion,* (291–308). Hillsdale, NJ: Lawrence Erlbaum Associates, 2003.

McKinley, N. M., & Randa, L. A. "Adult attachment and body satisfaction: An exploration of general and specific relationship differences." *Body Image, 2* (2005): 209–218.

O'Kearney, R. "Attachment disruption in anorexia nervosa and bulimia nervosa: A review of theory and empirical research." *International Journal of Eating Disorders, 20* (1996): 115–127.

[6] Fernandez, S., & Pritchard, M. "Relationships between self-esteem, media influence and drive for thinness." *Eating Behaviors, 13* (2012): 321-325. doi:10.1016/j.eatbeh.2012.05.004

[7] Tucci, S., & Peters, J. "Media influences on body dissatisfaction in female students." *Psicothema, 20*(4) (2008): 521–524.

[8] Ahern, A. L., Bennett, K. M., & Hetherington, M. M. "Internalization of the ultra-thin ideal: Positive implicit associations with underweight fashion models are associated with drive for thinness in young women." *Eating Disorders: The Journal of Treatment & Prevention, 16*(4) (2008): 294–307, http://dx.doi.org/10.1080/10640260802115852.

Harrison, K., & Cantor, J. "The relationship between media consumption and eating disorders." *Journal of Communication*, 47(1) (1997): 40–67, http://dx.doi.org/ 10.1111/j.1460-2466.1997. tb02692.x.

Hobza, C. L., Walker, K. E., Yakushko, O., & Peugh, J. L. "What about men? Social comparison and the effects of media images on body and self-esteem." *Psychology of Men & Masculinity*, 8(3) (2007): 161–172, http://dx.doi.org/10.1037/1524-9220.8.3.161.

Thomsen, S. R., Weber, M. M., & Beth Brown, L. "The relationship between reading beauty and fashion magazines and the use of pathogenic dieting methods among adolescent females." *Adolescence*, 37(145) (2002b): 1–18.

Wright, A., & Pritchard, M. E. "An examination of the relation of gender, mass media influences, and loneliness to disordered eating among college students." *Eating and Weight Disorders*, 14(2–3) (2009): e144–e147.

9   Hobza, C. L., & Rochlen, A. B. "Gender role conflict, drive for muscularity, and the impact of ideal media portrayals on men." *Psychology of Men & Masculinity*, 10(2) (2009): 120–130, http:// dx.doi.org/10.1037/a0015040.

Hobza, C. L., Walker, K. E., Yakushko, O., & Peugh, J. L. "What about men? Social comparison and the effects of media images on body and self-esteem." *Psychology of Men & Masculinity*, 8(3) (2007):161–172, http://dx.doi.org/10.1037/1524-9220.8.3.161.

Wright, A., & Pritchard, M. E. "An examination of the relation of gender, mass media influences, and loneliness to disordered eating among college students." *Eating and Weight Disorders, 14*(2–3) (2009): e144–e147.

10   Holmqvist, K. & Frisén, A. " 'I bet they aren't that perfect in reality': Appearance ideals viewed from the perspective of adolescents with a positive body image." *Body Image, 9* (2012): 388-395. http://dx.doi.org/10.1016/j.bodyim.2012.03.007

11   American Psychological Association, Task Force on the Sexualization of Girls. (2010). *Report of the APA Task Force on the Sexualization of Girls.* Retrieved from http://www.apa.org/pi/women/programs/girls/report-full.pdf.

12   Abraczinskas, M., Fisak, B., & Barnes, R. "The relation between parental influence, body image, and eating behaviors in a nonclinical female sample." *Body Image: An International Journal of Research, 9* (2012): 93-100. doi:10.1016/j.bodyim.2011.10.005

Ogden, J., & Steward, J. "The role of the mother-daughter relationship in explaining weight concern." *The International Journal of Eating Disorders, 28*(1) (2000): 78-83.

Smolak, L., Levine, M., & Schermer, F. "Parental input and weight concerns among elementary school children." *International Journal of Eating Disorders, 25* (1999): 263–271.

13   Wolf, N. *The Beauty Myth: How Images of Female Beauty Are Used Against Women.* New York, NY: William Morrow, 1991.

14   American Psychological Association, Task Force on the Sexualization of Girls. (2010). *Report of the APA Task Force on the*

Sexualization of Girls. Retrieved from http://www.apa.org/pi/
women/programs/girls/report-full.pdf.

15   Irving, L., & Berel, S. R. "Comparison of media-literacy programs to
strengthen college women's resistance to media images." *Psychology
of Women Quarterly, 5* (2001): 103-112.

16   Irving, L. M., DuPen, J., & Berel, S. "A media literacy program for
high school females." *Eating Disorders: The Journal of Treatment and
Prevention, 6* (1998): 119-132.

17   Cook, D.T., & Kaiser, S. B. "Betwixt and between: Age ambiguity
and the sexualization of the female consuming subject." *Journal of
Consumer Culture, 4* (2004): 203-227.

18   Kilbourne, J. *Deadly Persuasion: Why Women and Girls Must Fight the
Addictive Power of Advertising.* New York: Free Press, 1999.

American Psychological Association, Task Force on the
Sexualization of Girls. (2010). *Report of the APA Task Force on the
Sexualization of Girls.* Retrieved from http://www.apa.org/pi/
women/programs/girls/report-full.pdf

19   Duffy, M., & Gotcher, J. M. "Crucial advice on how to get the guy:
The rhetorical vision of power and seduction in the teen magazine
YM." *Journal of Communication Inquiry, 20* (1996): 32-48.

20   www.fightthenewdrug.org

21   Quigg, S.L., & Want, S.C. "Highlighting media modifications: Can a
television commercial mitigate the effects of music videos on female

appearance satisfaction?" *Body Image: An International Journal of Research,* 8 (2011): 135-142. doi:10.1016/j.bodyim.2010.11.008

22 Piran, N., & Teall, T. "The Developmental Theory of Embodiment." In G. McVey, M. P. Levine, N. Piran, & H. B. Ferguson (Eds.), *Preventing Eating-Related and Weight-Related Disorders: Collaborative Research, Advocacy, and Policy Change* (pp. 171-199). Waterloo, ON: Wilfred Laurier Press, 2012.

23 Ibid.

24 Gilligan, C. *In a different voice: Psychological Theory and Women's Development.* Cambridge, MA: Harvard University Press, 1982.

25 Anda, R. F., Felitti, V. J., Bremner, J. D., Walker, J. D., Whitfield, C. H., Perry, B. D., ... & Giles, W. H. "The enduring effects of abuse and related adverse experiences in childhood." *European Archives of Psychiatry and Clinical Neuroscience,* 256(3) (2006): 174-186.

Brown, D. W., Anda, R. F., Tiemeier, H., Felitti, V. J., Edwards, V. J., Croft, J. B., & Giles, W. H. "Adverse childhood experiences and the risk of premature mortality." *American Journal of Preventive Medicine,* 37(5) (2009): 389-396.

Chapman, D. P., Whitfield, C. L., Felitti, V. J., Dube, S. R., Edwards, V. J., & Anda, R. F. "Adverse childhood experiences and the risk of depressive disorders in adulthood." *Journal of Affective Disorders,* 82(2) (2004): 217-225.

Danese, A., Moffitt, T. E., Harrington, H., Milne, B. J., Polanczyk, G., Pariante, C. M., ... & Caspi, A. "Adverse childhood experiences and adult risk factors for age-related disease: depression, inflammation, and clustering of metabolic risk markers." *Archives of Pediatrics & Adolescent Medicine, 163*(12) (2009): 1135-1143.

Dube, S. R., Anda, R. F., Felitti, V. J., Chapman, D. P., Williamson, D. F., & Giles, W. H. "Childhood abuse, household dysfunction, and the risk of attempted suicide throughout the life span: Findings from the Adverse Childhood Experiences Study." *Jama, 286*(24) (2001): 3089-3096.

Dube, S. R., Felitti, V. J., Dong, M., Giles, W. H., & Anda, R. F. "The impact of adverse childhood experiences on health problems: evidence from four birth cohorts dating back to 1900." *Preventive Medicine, 37*(3) (2003): 268-277.

Felitti, V. J., & Anda, R. F. "The relationship of adverse childhood experiences to adult medical disease, psychiatric disorders and sexual behavior: Implications for healthcare." In *The impact of Early Life Trauma on Health and Disease: The Hidden Epidemic.* 77-87. Cambridge (UK) University Press.

Nakazawa, D. J. *Childhood Disrupted: How Your Biography Becomes Your Biology, and How You Can Heal.* New York, NY: Simon and Schuster, 2015.

Schilling, E. A., Aseltine, R. H., & Gore, S. "Adverse childhood experiences and mental health in young adults: a longitudinal survey." *BMC Public Health, 7*(1) (2007): 1.

[26] Levine, P. & Frederick, A. *Waking the Tiger: Healing Trauma* Berkeley, CA.: North Atlantic Books.

27   Brown, L. M. and Gilligan, C. *Meeting at the Crossroads: Women's Psychology and Girls' Development.* Cambridge, MA: Harvard University Press, 1992.

Gilligan, C. *In a Different Voice: Psychological Theory and Women's Development.* Cambridge, MA: Harvard University Press, 1982.

28   Miller, J. B. *The development of women's sense of self.* In Judith Jordan (Ed), Women's growth in connection: Writings from the Stone Center. (1991). New York, NY: Guilford, **THIS IS INCOMPLETE**

29   Brown, L. M. and Gilligan, C. *Meeting at the Crossroads: Women's Psychology and Girls' Development.* Cambridge, MA: Harvard University Press, 1992.

Buchholz, A. and White, D.R. *Relational authenticity, appearance esteem, and disordered eating in adolescent girls.* Poster presented at ISSBD, Quebec City, Canada.

Buchholz, A., Henderson, K. A., Hounsell, A., Wagner, A., Norris, M., & Spettigue, W. "Self-silencing in a clinical sample of female adolescents with eating disorders." *Journal of the Canadian Academy of Child and Adolescent Psychiatry,* 16(4) (2007): 158-163.

30   Buchholz, A., Henderson, K. A., Hounsell, A., Wagner, A., Norris, M., & Spettigue, W. "Self-silencing in a clinical sample of female adolescents with eating disorders." *Journal of the Canadian Academy of Child and Adolescent Psychiatry,* 16(4) (2007): 158-163.

31   Jack, D. C. *Silencing the Self: Women and Depression.* Cambridge, MA: Harvard University Press, 1991.

[32] Gilligan, C. "Adolescent development reconsidered." In C. Gilligan, J. Ward & A. J. Tayler (Eds.). *Mapping the Moral Domain*. Boston, MA: Harvard University Press, 1988.

[33] Fredrickson, B. L., & Roberts, T. "Objectification theory: Toward understanding women's lived experiences and mental health risks." *Psychology of Women Quarterly*, *21* (1997): 173-206.

[34] Piran, N., & Teall, T. "The Developmental Theory of Embodiment." In G. McVey, M. P. Levine, N. Piran, & H. B. Ferguson, *Preventing Eating-Related and Weight-Related Disorders: Collaborative Research, Advocacy, and Policy Change* (pp. 171-199). Waterloo, ON: Wilfred Laurier Press, 2012.

[35] Murnen, S. K., & Smolak, L. "Are feminist women protected from body image problems? A meta-analytic review of relevant research." *Sex Roles*, *60* (2009): 186-197.

[36] Piran, N., & Teall, T. "The Developmental Theory of Embodiment." In G. McVey, M. P. Levine, N. Piran, & H. B. Ferguson, *Preventing Eating-Related and Weight-Related Disorders: Collaborative Research, Advocacy, and Policy Change*. 171-199. Waterloo ON: Wilfred Laurier Press, 2012.

[37] Elium, J. & Elium, D. *Raising a Daughter: Parents and the Awakening of a Healthy Woman*. 34. New York, NY: Random House, 2003.

[38] Ibid, pg 135.

[39] Mask, L., & Blanchard, C. M. "The protective role of general self-determination against 'thin ideal' media exposure on women's body

image and eating-related concerns." *Journal of Health psychology,* *16*(3) (2011): 489-499.

[40] Brown, C., Weber, S., & Ali, S. "Women's body talk: A Feminist Narrative approach." *Journal of Systemic Therapies,* 27 (2) (2008): 92-104.

[41] Brownmiller, S. *Femininity.* New York, NY: Fawcett Columbine, 1984.

Martin, C. E. *Perfect Girls, Starving Daughters: The Frightening New Normalcy of Hating Your Body.* New York, NY: Simon and Schuster, 2007. Wolf, N. *The Beauty Myth.* New York, NY: Chatto and Windus, 1991.

[42] MacKnee, C. M. "Profound sexual and spiritual encounters among practicing Christians: A phenomenological analysis." *Journal of Psychology and Theology,* 30(3) (2002): 234.

[43] Melton, G.D. *Carry On, Warrior: The Power of Embracing Your Messy, Beautiful Life.* New York, NY: Scribner, 2014.

[44] Siegel, D. *The Developing Mind: How Relationships and the Brain Interact to Shape Who We Are.* New York, NY: Guilford Press, 2015.

[45] American Psychological Association, Task Force on the Sexualization of Girls. (2010). *Report of the APA Task Force on the Sexualization of Girls.* Retrieved from http://www.apa.org/pi/women/programs/girls/report-full.pdf

[46] Brumariu, L. E. "Parent–Child attachment and emotion regulation." *New Directions for Child and Adolescent Development,* 2015(148) 2015: 31-45. doi:10.1002/cad.20098

Kim, B., Stifter, C. A., Philbrook, L. E., & Teti, D. M. "Infant emotion regulation: Relations to bedtime emotional availability, attachment security, and temperament." *Infant Behavior & Development,* 37(4) (2014): 480-490. doi:10.1016/j. infbeh.2014.06.006

Morris, A. S., Silk, J. S., Steinberg, L., Myers, S. S., & Robinson, L. R. "The role of the family context in the development of emotion regulation." *Social Development,* 16(2) (2007): 361-388. doi:10.1111/j.1467-9507.2007.00389.x

Schore, A. N. *Affect Regulation and the Origin of the Self: The Neurobiology of Emotional Development.* Hillsdale, N.J: L. Erlbaum Associates, 1994.

Schore, A. N. "Back to basics: Attachment, affect regulation, and the developing right brain: Linking developmental neuroscience to pediatrics." *Pediatrics in Review,* 26(6) (2005): 204-217. doi:10.1542/pir.26-6-204

Schore, A. N. *Affect Regulation and the Origin of the Self: The Neurobiology of Emotional Development.* Abingdon: Psychology Press, 2015. doi:10.4324/9781315680019

Schore, J. R., & Schore, A. N. "Modern attachment theory: The central role of affect regulation in development and treatment." *Clinical Social Work Journal,* 36(1) (2008): 9-20. doi:10.1007/ s10615-007-0111-7

Spangler, G., & Zimmermann, P. "Emotional and adrenocortical regulation in early adolescence: Prediction by attachment security and disorganization in infancy." *International*

Journal of Behavioral Development, 38(2) (2014): 142-154. doi:10.1177/0165025414520808

47   Brumariu, L. E. "Parent–Child attachment and emotion regulation." New Directions for Child and Adolescent Development, 2015(148) (2015): 31-45. doi:10.1002/cad.20098

Bialik, M. Beyond the Sling: A Real-Life Guide to Raising Confident, Loving Children the Attachment Parenting Way. New York, NY: Touchstone, 2012.

Morris, A. S., Silk, J. S., Steinberg, L., Myers, S. S., & Robinson, L. R. "The role of the family context in the development of emotion regulation." Social Development, 16(2) (2007): 361-388. doi:10.1111/j.1467-9507.2007.00389.x

Schore, A. N. Affect Regulation and the Origin of the Self: The Neurobiology of Emotional Development. Hillsdale, N.J: L. Erlbaum Associates, 1994.

Schore, A. N. "Back to basics: Attachment, affect regulation, and the developing right brain: Linking developmental neuroscience to pediatrics." Pediatrics in Review, 26(6) (2005): 204-217. doi:10.1542/pir.26-6-204

Schore, A. N. Affect Regulation and the Origin of the Self: The Neurobiology of Emotional Development. Abingdon: Psychology Press. doi:10.4324/9781315680019

Schore, J. R., & Schore, A. N. "Modern attachment theory: The central role of affect regulation in development and treatment."

Clinical Social Work Journal, 36(1) (2008): 9-20. doi:10.1007/s10615-007-0111-7

Spangler, G., & Zimmermann, P. "Emotional and adrenocortical regulation in early adolescence: Prediction by attachment security and disorganization in infancy." *International Journal of Behavioral Development*, 38(2) (2014): 142-154. doi:10.1177/0165025414520808

[48] http://emotion.utu.fi

Nummenmaa, L., Glerean, E., Hari, R., & Hietanen, J. K. "Bodily maps of emotions." *Proceedings of the National Academy of Sciences*, 111(2) (2014): 646 - 651. doi:10.1073/pnas.1321664111

[49] Damasio, A. *The Feeling of What Happens: Body and Emotion in the Making of Consciousness.* Boston, MA: Mariner Books, 1999.

[50] I'm using the word "learned" here to reflect both intentional and unintentional (modeling) messages we've experienced, or observed in others close to us.

[51] Bradley, S. J. *Affect Regulation and the Development of Psychopathology.* New York, NY: Guilford Press, 2000.

Bresin, K., & Gordon, K. H. "Endogenous opioids and nonsuicidal self-injury: A mechanism of affect regulation." *Neuroscience and Biobehavioral Reviews*, 37(3) (2013): 374-383. doi:10.1016/j.neubiorev.2013.01.020

Eftekhari, A., Zoellner, L. A., & Vigil, S. A. "Patterns of emotion regulation and psychopathology." *Anxiety, Stress & Coping*, 22(5) (2009): 571-586. doi:10.1080/10615800802179860

Gross, J. J., & Jazaieri, H. "Emotion, emotion regulation, and psychopathology: An affective science perspective." *Clinical Psychological Science*, 2(4) (2014): 387-401. doi:10.1177/2167702614536164

Tasca, G. A., Szadkowski, L., Illing, V., Trinneer, A., Grenon, R., Demidenko, N., . . . Bissada, H. ("Adult attachment, depression, and eating disorder symptoms: The mediating role of affect regulation strategies." *Personality and Individual Differences*, 47(6) (2009): 662-667. doi:10.1016/j.paid.2009.06.006

Brockmeyer, T., Skunde, M., Wu, M., Bresslein, E., Rudofsky, G., Herzog, W., & Friederich, H. "Difficulties in emotion regulation across the spectrum of eating disorders." *Comprehensive Psychiatry*, 55(3) (2014): 565- 571. doi:10.1016/j.comppsych.2013.12.001

Harrison, A., Sullivan, S., Tchanturia, K., & Treasure, J. "Emotional functioning in eating disorders: Attentional bias, emotion recognition and emotion regulation." *Psychological Medicine*, 40(11) (2010): 1887-1897. doi:10.1017/S0033291710000036

Harrison, C., Mitchison, D., Rieger, E., Rodgers, B., & Mond, J. "Emotion regulation difficulties in binge eating disorder with and without the overvaluation of weight and shape." *Psychiatry Research*, 245 (2016): 436-442. doi:10.1016/j.psychres.2016.09.005

Haynos, A. F., Roberto, C. A., & Attia, E. "Examining the associations between emotion regulation difficulties, anxiety, and eating disorder severity among inpatients with anorexia nervosa." *Comprehensive Psychiatry*, 60 (2015): 93-98. doi:10.1016/j.comppsych.2015.03.004

Lavender, J. M., Wonderlich, S. A., Peterson, C. B., Crosby, R. D., Engel, S. G., Mitchell, J. E., . . . Berg, K. C. "Dimensions of emotion dysregulation in bulimia nervosa." *European Eating Disorders Review*, 22(3) (2014): 212-216. doi:10.1002/erv.2288

Naumann, E., Tuschen-Caffier, B., Voderholzer, U., & Svaldi, J. "Spontaneous emotion regulation in anorexia and bulimia nervosa." *Cognitive Therapy and Research*, 40(3) (2016): 304-313. doi:10.1007/s10608-015-9723-3

Rowsell, M., MacDonald, D. E., & Carter, J. C. "Emotion regulation difficulties in anorexia nervosa: Associations with improvements in eating psychopathology." *Journal of Eating Disorders*, 4 (2016): 17. doi: 10.1186/s40337-016-0108-0

ABOUT THE AUTHOR

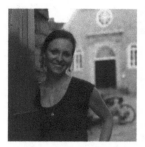

Hillary McBride is a PhD candidate at the University of British Columbia in Counselling Psychology. In her doctoral studies, she is continuing research she started in her masters studies exploring women's experiences in and of the body, particularly at significant transitions or points of development. McBride owns a private practice in Vancouver, BC, where she sees adults and couples for a variety of concerns, including acute mental health issues. She works regularly with people struggling with depression, anxiety, life transitions, self-harm, abuse, relationship issues, and sexuality. She specializes in women's issues from a feminist perspective (including perinatal mental health, body image, and disordered eating) as well as trauma and trauma therapies for ongoing childhood abuse to single incident adult trauma. She designed and conducted body image presentations and groups for young girls and their mothers that she presents regularly in schools and community settings. Hillary now serves on the board of directors for Free to Be, and speaks regularly on radio, podcasts, and at workshops on a variety of mental health topics including sexuality, body image, well-being, living authentically, and healing trauma.

In addition to being an academic and clinician who specializes in these issues, McBride is a survivor of an eating disorder, with which she struggled and received formal treatment for many years. As part of her healing journey, she made a commitment to learn more about what contributed to the development of the disorder in her life, and to find ways to create a world in which girls and women no longer have to struggle in the same way.

McBride enjoys spending time with her husband, riding her bike, playing guitar and violin, drinking chai, and finding ways to contribute to her community.